Discover Superfoods #1

21 Best Superfood Cacao Recipes

"Cacao is Nature's Healthy and Delicious
Superfood Chocolate you can enjoy even on
a weight loss or low cholesterol diet."

Donna Davidson

&

Kay Wood

DISCLAIMER

Any references to the health benefits of superfood ingredients in
this recipe book are the opinions of the authors, based on the best data
currently available to them, and are provided for informational
purposes only; they are not intended as medical advice.

If you have an existing medical condition and/or concerns about eating
any of the ingredients mentioned in this book, you should seek the
advice of a qualified medical practitioner before doing so.

Serving Sizes

Serving sizes indicated in this book are intended as a guide only.
Actual serving sizes often vary between individuals,
so feel free to alter them to suit your self.

* * *

ISBN: 978-0-473-36727-5

THANK YOU GIFT
FROM DONNA & KAY

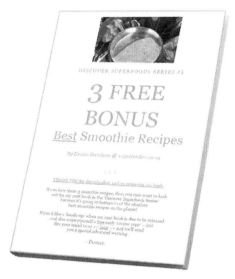

As a reward for getting our book, we'd like to give you

3 FREE SMOOTHIE RECIPES

[Yes, Superfood Smoothies!]

They're a taste of our 2nd book,
21 Best Superfood Smoothie Recipes
- Discover Superfoods #2 - now on Amazon.com

<< GET YOUR FREE RECIPES HERE >>

Type this into your Internet browser:
www.superfoodies.co.nz/book1free

We think you'll like them!

Milking the Cacao?

Can, so-called, 'superfoods' really help you be healthier and feel better?

Good question.

I'm often asked things like, "Can learning to make chocolate recipes (of all things!), using a costlier raw, organic version of chocolate *really* be so much better for you?"

Or, "Can Cacao and the other, so-called, 'superfoods' seriously contribute to a low-cholesterol diet, or help someone trying to achieve weight loss, or battle debilitating health problems?"

Well, that's *exactly* what happened to me.

Today, six years on from my first tentative superfoods experiments, I'm feeling better and healthier than I'd felt for years during my 'pre-superfoods' days. I'm not alone. Over the past six years, I discovered a talent for persuading superfood sceptics to try them, simply by relating my own story.

Most of these (now) former sceptics reported back to me of experiencing the same increased sense of well-being and improved mental acuity that I found. Over time, others experienced (often to their great joy) similar relief from persistent, debilitating health issues; which I had earlier achieved by the simple means of drinking a green superfood smoothie every morning for breakfast. I didn't change anything else in my diet at the time, either.

So, 'the proof is in the pudding', as they say.

In fact, I have a very special chocolate pudding in this very book for you to find it in! (Section B, Cacao Powder recipes, pg.30)

Since I began working in the superfoods industry, 6 years ago, I always used myself as a guinea pig for the products I sold. I never wanted someone else to put something into their body that I hadn't personally tested and could vouch for as both safe and effective. Initially, the main effect I noticed was increased energy levels and an improvement in my mental clarity.

I was happy enough with that. However, it got better.

Within 3 months, I also overcame health issues that I'd struggled with for years - in spite of being a very fit, active person, working in the sports / health and fitness industry for most of my life.

Today, just three years after starting an online superfoods business, (superfoodies.co.nz) I find myself helping satisfy a growing local demand for high quality dried superfoods, for New Zealand (where I live) and Australians. However, I recently received my first, and *very* substantial, order from Dubai! I don't know how they found me, as they didn't know about my website. The cost of shipping to Dubai didn't faze them either, so… a wealthy Saudi, keen to learn how to make a healthy Sheik? The word is definitely spreading.

This book (and the rest of the 'Discover Superfoods' series) is designed to be an easy introduction to superfoods; simple recipes, easy to make, tasting absolutely delicious.

If you got this book for *yourself*, you're either a 'superfoods newbie' looking for a place to start, or an existing superfoods fan looking new ideas. Either way, I wrote this book for you. Please dive in and enjoy each healthy chocolate recipe … guilt-free!

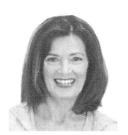

Your Very Good Health,

Donna

Donna Davidson
August, 2016.

Meet the Authors …

Donna Davidson

Now happily living by the Pacific Ocean in beautiful New Zealand, Donna's primary passion has always been in the health, fitness and well-being arena. Several years ago, while working in the superfoods industry, Donna personally experienced the profound benefits of incorporating superfoods into her regular diet and she now credits them with … Read more on pg.58

Kay Wood

Originally from the world of advertising and marketing, Kay has more recently specialised in copywriting and content creation for the Internet. For nearly 10 years Kay has been 'ghost-writing' info blogs for online businesses and offering her help to clients struggling to turn their awkward prose and bad spelling into simple and easily understood … Read more on pg.62

Meet the Real Cacao …

Health Benefits of Cacao: nature's organic chocolate.

Cacao is a raw, organic chocolate superfood. It contains high levels of the antioxidants, which are vital for protecting our cells and tissues from disease, and may help to slow cell degeneration. Cacao is also rich in … Read more on pg.56

What are Superfoods?

Superfoods are a special category of foods found in nature. These foods are superior sources of the anti-oxidants and essential nutrients that our bodies need, but cannot make themselves. Superfoods are calorie-sparse and nutrient-dense, so they pack a lot of punch for their weight and deliver … Read more on pg.64

Superfoods Descriptions + Info

Sacha Inchi Protein Powder: Vegetable protein powder from the South American Sacha Inchi seed. Contains 60% complete protein, all essential amino acids acids, as well as the omega essential fatty acids. Easily digestible and light nutty flavour. Perfect for pre and post workout smoothies, maintaining … Read more on pg.66

Testimonials about Superfoods

Lost over 7kg and feeling so much better: Thank you so much for the healthy delicious treats (see recipe pg.8) for Christmas. I am still enjoying my new eating regime with super foods. I have lost over 7kg and feeling so much better in myself. Everyone comments on how well I … Read more on pg.70

Meet the Real Proof …

Will, so-called, 'superfoods' really help me become healthier and feel better? Consider the vital relationship between our modern diet and our health: the steady and observable decline in health and rise of chronic conditions such as allergies, asthma, and skin conditions in western countries over the last 60-100 years is generally agreed, by scientists and … Read more on pg.84

Try the Chocolate Pudding Challenge …

The proof is in the pudding.

In our experience, most people find after adding superfoods to their regular diet (often by simply replacing breakfast with a 'superfood smoothie') that they feel more energetic, start noticing improvements or even the elimination of … Read full 'Chocolate Pudding Challenge' on pg.87

* * *

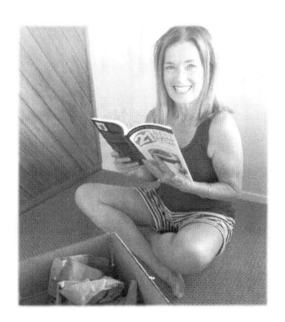

Dreaming of writing your own book?

Many people spend years wanting to write a book but never do ... Why?

How did _we_ manage it?

We found a great online writers group, called 'Self-Publishing School'.
They provided coaching, training, support, and a step-by-step plan
to publishing our first book in 90 days, guaranteed.

They also showed us how to format, upload, and successfully market
our book. They involved us in a supportive Facebook community
of fellow writers who gave immediate feedback and positive
advice all along the way. We had a great experience, and
our books have all made it to No.1 on Amazon,
so we happily commend SPS to you.

If you believe you have a book in you, but need
a little help giving birth to it, check out the
Self-Publishing School at the link below:

Self-Publishing School -
http://superfoodies.co.nz/sps

PHOTO Opposite left: The joy of a new author seeing her book in print for the first time!

Donna Davidson and Kay Wood

ACKNOWLEDGMENTS

Special Thanks to ::
Louise, Susie, Debs, and Anna
- for their wonderful recipe contributions.

A special thanks to :: the Self-Publishing School gang,
especially Chandler Bolt and Sean Sumner. Without your
amazing coaching and easy step-by-step plan, this book
would probably never exist. We are indebted to you.

We totally recommend Self-Publishing School:
http://superfoodies.co.nz/sps

Photo Contributors :: Maaka McQuillan, Jess Thomson
Graphic Design, Layout, Copywriting :: Kay Wood
Recipe Creation + Testing :: Donna Davidson
Kindle eBook Formatting :: Jay Syder

Published by ::
Super Healthy Kiwi Publishing

Contact the authors by Snail Mail ::
SuperFoodies NZ
267a Harbour Road
Ohope Beach 3121
New Zealand

Email :: info@superfoodies.co.nz
Website :: http://superfoodies.co.nz
Facebook :: facebook.com/superfoodies.co.nz

x

Table of Contents

WHERE TO START?

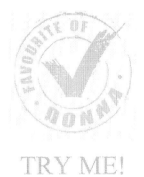

TRY ME!

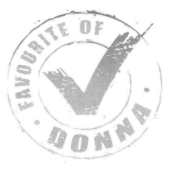

Not sure which recipe to try <u>first</u>?

They all look good, right?

We've made it easy for you. We'll give you a 'tick start'.
The above 'tick' icon appears next to 3 personally
chosen recipes, one from each cacao section.

<u>Donna's Top 3</u>
'Tick Start' Recipes!

1. **Chocolate Caramel Slice** >>> TRY ME on pg.2
2. **Blueberry Chocolate Mousse Torte** >>> TRY ME on pg.26
3. **Maqui Berry Cacao Truffles** >>> TRY ME on pg.42

Each, is a <u>great</u> first choice.

"Why not pick a top 3 recipe and try it tonight? I know
you'll find it delicious, energising, and much
better for you and your loved ones."

−Donna.

PS.

Choosing my 'Top 3' was genuine agony (Kay forced me!),
because I love *all* the recipes in this book.

Donna Davidson and Kay Wood

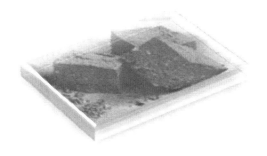

SECTION A

CACAO

BUTTER

recipes

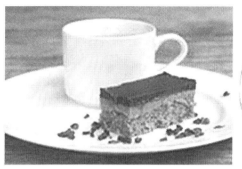 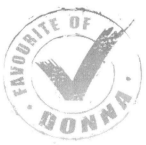

A1. Chocolate Caramel Slice

Serving size: makes 30 slices
Time to make: 35 minutes

Base Ingredients

2½ cups walnuts
½ cup dried dates - soaked for 15 minutes in hot water
1 cup desiccated coconut
2 tablespoons lucuma powder
½ teaspoon vanilla paste
1 pinch of salt
¼ teaspoon ground cinnamon
1 tablespoon maple syrup / or yacon syrup

Caramel Ingredients

½ cup almond butter
1 tablespoon lucuma powder
1 pinch of salt
½ teaspoon vanilla paste
1 cup liquid coconut oil
¼ cup maple syrup / or yacon syrup

Chocolate Topping Ingredients

130g cacao butter
$\frac{1}{3}$ cup cacao powder
1 tablespoon honey
$\frac{1}{4}$ cup maple syrup / or yacon syrup

Base Method

1. Blitz walnuts in blender until nice and fine (but not powder). Set aside.
2. Make a date paste in the blender with the soaked dates and add some date water if needed to make a smooth sticky paste.
3. Return nuts to the blender with all other base ingredients and blitz until well combined. You can finish off combining with your hands, if you find that easier.
4. Line a medium size slice tin with baking paper and press in the base mixture. Once evenly flattened put in refrigerator or freezer while you make the caramel.

Caramel Method

1. Before starting, make sure that the almond butter is at room temperature, and the coconut oil isn't too hot – it should be just warm enough to be liquid.
2. Place almond butter, lucuma, salt, vanilla paste and maple syrup in blender. Mix on low until smooth, then slowly pour in the coconut oil.
3. Once all oil is added, blitz on high speed until well combined and smooth.
4. Pour this caramel mixture evenly over the base and return to the refrigerator / or freezer to set, before making the chocolate topping.

Chocolate Topping Method

1. Melt cacao butter in bowl placed in a larger bowl filled with boiling water. Once melted add all other ingredients and whisk with a hand whisk.
2. Pour chocolate on top of caramel and return to fridge.
3. After about 15 minutes and (very important) before the chocolate sets 'hard', remove from the refrigerator and 'score' some cutting lines into the chocolate with a sharp knife. If you neglect this step the chocolate topping will splinter when cutting into slices later on. Return to refrigerator to set completely.
4. When fully set, remove from the refrigerator and cut into slices along your previous 'score' lines with a sharp knife. Garnish with a sprinkle of cacao nibs and serve.

* Notes:

TIP: If you melt your cacao butter first, then it will be ready when you need it.

This Chocolate Caramel Slice will keep in the refrigerator for about 2 weeks, or indefinitely in the freezer.

The serving size of 30 slices obviously depends on how *big* you like your slices - so please take my serving size indications as a guide only, and slice the pieces to suit yourself.

NEXT Cacao Butter recipe:
| A2 | Orange Chocolate Fudge | Pg.6

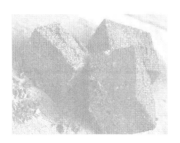

"Cacao is high in the antioxidants we need
to help keep our cells healthy."

-Donna.

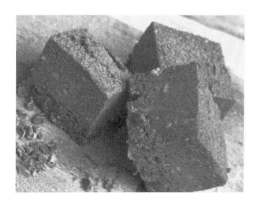

A2. Orange Chocolate Fudge

Serving size: makes 48 pieces
Time to make: 30 minutes

Base Ingredients

¼ cup cacao powder
1 cup walnuts
½ cup coconut
¼ cup cacao nibs
½ cup dried dates - soaked in hot water for approx. 15 minutes
1 tablespoon tahini
1 tablespoon lucuma powder / or yacon powder

Topping Ingredients

100g cacao butter
2 oranges - rind and juice
2½ cups raw cashew nuts
½ cup maple syrup / or yacon syrup
¾ cup cacao powder

Base Method

1. Blitz walnuts in blender until they are a rough powder, then put aside until needed.

2. Soak the dates (12 dates is about ½ cup) in boiling water for 15 minutes. Make a date paste by blending the dates in the blender and adding the date water until you get a nice sticky smooth paste.

3. Add all base ingredients to the blender and blitz until well mixed. Remove from blender and mix by hand if needed. Press into a 26cm x 19cm dish lined with baking paper.

4. Place in refrigerator, or freezer, for 30 minutes - or while you are making the filling.

Topping Method

1. Blitz cashew nuts into a fine powder.

2. Melt cacao butter (Note: Cacao butter is easy to burn if you melt it in a pot on the stove. I always stand it in a dish sitting in a larger dish of boiling water for 15 minutes.)

3. Place all topping ingredients in blender, with cashew nut powder, and mix together until smooth.

4. Remove base from refrigerator and spread the fudge mixture on top.

5. Return to refrigerator to set. Setting takes 30-60 minutes.

* Notes:

Your fudge will be easier to cut up if you remember to 'score' it just before it fully sets. It will keep in the refrigerator for up to 2 weeks. You can also freeze it, to keep it longer.

NEXT Cacao Butter recipe:
| A3 | Christmas 'Black Forest' Chocolate Treats | Pg.8

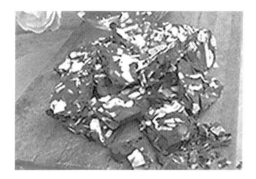

A3. Christmas Black Forest Chocolate Treats

Serving size: makes 50 pieces
Time to make: 15 minutes

I've created this quick and very easy 'black forest treats' recipe to help make your Christmas chocolate snacking a whole lot healthier – but still appropriately yummy.

Ingredients

1 cup cacao butter
½ cup cacao powder
½ cup yacon powder / or ¼ cup coconut nectar / or maple syrup / or honey
¼ cup coconut chips
2 tablespoons goji berries
2 tablespoons pepitas (pumpkin seeds)
2 tablespoons dried cranberries / or dried fruit of your choice

Method

1. Place cacao butter into a heat-proof bowl over a pot of slowly simmering water to melt. I sit the bowl in the top section of a 'double boiler' saucepan.

2. Remove from heat and use a whisk to beat in the cacao and yacon powders, or sweetener, until dissolved.

3. Pour liquid chocolate mix into a 24x19 cm baking dish lined with baking paper and sprinkle the coconut, goji berries, pepitas and dried cranberries, or other dried fruit, over the top.

4. Place in the freezer for 10-30 minutes to set. Once the chocolate is set, break into pieces.

* Notes:

This Christmas you can treat your friends and family to this healthy chocolate superfood snack that is 'calorie friendly' - yet still packed with all the decadent indulgence they expect.

If you want your chocolate pieces to be 'uniform' in size, then you will need to 'score' the chocolate with a sharp knife before it completely sets. Otherwise, you will be looking at it breaking up into a variety of irregular shapes - which can be fun too. Although, maybe not if you have children (or a spouse) who like to fight over who gets the biggest piece!

NEXT Cacao Butter recipe:
| A4 | Healthy Homemade Chocolates | Pg.10

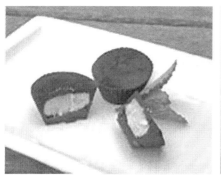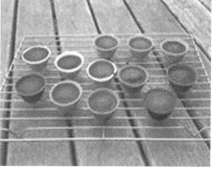

A4. Healthy Homemade Chocolates

Serving size: makes 12 chocolates
Time to make: 30 minutes

This recipe for healthy, homemade chocolates is easy and the results look spectacular. As an amateur chocolate maker, I couldn't believe my eyes when first I watched them emerge from their molds looking so 'professionally-made'. They taste absolutely delicious too! You'll need 12 mini molds (I like the new silicon ones) to create the chocolate shapes.

Ingredients - for chocolate outsides

30g cacao butter
½ cup cacao powder
2 teaspoons coconut nectar / or brown rice malt syrup / or maple syrup
3 tablespoons extra virgin coconut oil

Ingredients - for chocolate centres

3 tablespoons coconut butter (see notes below to make your own)
1 drop of peppermint essential oil - culinary-grade
½ teaspoon coconut nectar

2 tablespoons extra virgin coconut oil

Method

1. Place the coconut oil and cacao butter in a bowl to melt. Place this bowl in a bigger dish of boiling water to melt, or if you prefer melt over a saucepan of boiling water.
2. Once melted, take the bowl out of the water and add the cacao powder and coconut nectar. Pour into a jug.
3. Arrange 12 mini silicon cups on a tray and fill each case with chocolate (enough to fill the base of the cup). Place the tray in the fridge or freezer to set (takes about 10 minutes).
4. In the meantime, return the remaining chocolate mixture left over in the jug back to the hot water dish to keep it liquefied.

Method - for the centres

1. Place all centre ingredients in a bowl and melt over hot water just enough to combine ingredients and have a firm manageable mixture, don't melt to a liquid.
2. Divide into 12 equal amounts or measure a teaspoon full and mould into a flattened ball.
3. Take chocolate base out of the fridge and place the filling in the centre of each cup. Return to fridge or freezer to set.
4. When nicely firm, take out of freezer and pour the remaining chocolate into each case. Remember to leave enough space around the peppermint centre for the chocolate to run down the sides.

* Notes:

How to make your own Coconut Butter (optional)

Coconut Butter Ingredients

1 cup of shredded or desiccated coconut

1 teaspoon melted extra-virgin coconut oil

1 pinch of salt

Coconut Butter Method

1. Place the coconut in a blender and blitz on high speed, until it becomes a butter consistency, this takes a couple of minutes.
2. Add some salt and coconut oil to adjust the texture (only if necessary) as you go.

You are aiming to make a nice *buttery paste*. If you think that the paste has become a little too runny, keep in mind that it will become thicker again when you rest it.

NEXT Cacao Butter recipe:
| A5 | Peanut Butter Squares | Pg.14

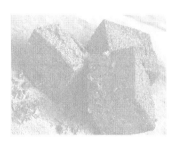

"Cacao is a mood elevator due to
the presence of serotonin."

-Donna.

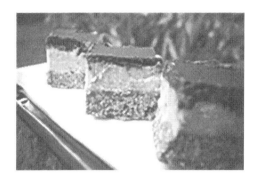

A5. Peanut Butter Squares

Serving size: makes 24 squares
Time to make: 30 minutes

Base Ingredients

3 tablespoons honey
5 tablespoons peanut butter
1 tablespoon cacao powder
2 tablespoons cacao nibs
1 cup desiccated coconut

Centre Ingredients

3 tablespoons honey
6 tablespoons peanut butter
3 tablespoons coconut oil

Topping Ingredients

60g cacao butter
1 tablespoon honey
1 tablespoon maple syrup
1½ tablespoons cacao powder

Base Method

1. Place honey and peanut butter into a medium sized bowl and mix to combine. (Warm the peanut butter and honey slightly - so they will mix easily)
2. Add cacao powder and nibs and mix to combine. Then add coconut and mix again.
3. Use hands to work the mixture, until it is sticking together.
4. Press mixture firmly into 20 x 10 cm loaf tin lined with baking paper.
5. Place in refrigerator to set.

Centre Method

1. Place ingredients into a saucepan and heat over very low heat until the mixture has just softened and the oil melted.
2. Remove from heat and mix until smooth and well combined.
3. Pour mixture over base and place in fridge or freezer to set.

Topping Method

1. It is best to wait until the middle layer is set before making the topping, but it doesn't take long. Place cacao butter in a heat proof bowl, sit bowl in boiling water so cacao butter can melt.
2. When totally melted, remove bowl from water dish and add the honey, maple syrup and cacao powder.
3. Mix well with whisk, and pour chocolate topping over the middle layer.
4. Return to refrigerator to set.
5. Before mix has totally set (after about 10 minutes) remove from refrigerator and 'score' the chocolate topping into squares; otherwise the chocolate will split if you try to cut it when totally set hard. Return to refrigerator to set firmly.

* Notes:

For all the peanut butter lovers out there, this recipe truly is a treat. My friend Louise sent it to me because her children – the toughest food critics out there - absolutely love it and she wanted to share it with as many people as possible.

I added some cacao nibs to the base for a little extra chocolate 'hit' and increased antioxidant boost.

NEXT Cacao Butter recipe:
| A6 | Choc Fudge Protein Bar | Pg.18

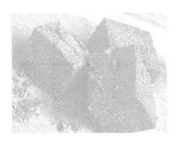

"Cacao is high in magnesium - an important mineral required for heart health."

-Donna.

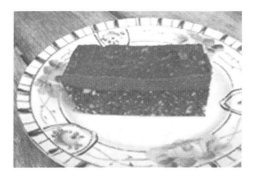

A6. Choc Fudge Protein Bar

Serving size: makes 30 bars
Time to make: 30 minutes

The great thing about this protein bar is that, as well as being packed full of protein and truly satisfying, you can still eat it 'guilt-free' because of its wonderfully healthy ingredients.

Base Ingredients

3 tablespoons cacao powder
1½ cup dried dates (dried dates need to be soaked to soften them)
½ cup desiccated coconut
1 cup almonds
1 cup almond flour
3 tablespoons sacha inchi protein powder
1 tablespoon maqui berry powder
2 teaspoons ginger powder
2 teaspoons cinnamon powder
2 tablespoons chia seeds
3 tablespoons lucuma powder
6 tablespoons melted coconut oil

Icing Ingredients

2 tablespoons cacao powder

¼ cup melted cacao butter

1 cup cashew nuts

¼ cup melted coconut oil

½ teaspoon vanilla paste

¼ cup maple syrup

¼ cup dates

Base Method

1. Soak dates in hot water to cover and leave for 15 minutes.
2. Pulse almonds in food processor, then place in a bowl with all the other dry ingredients.
3. Blitz dates in blender or food processor; use some of the date water to make a sticky paste - but also save some of the date water for later.
4. Add coconut oil to date paste and blend; add this mixture to the dry ingredients.
5. Mix with spoon or hands, adding date water if necessary. It needs to be cohesive enough to form a single 'ball' using all the mixture.
6. Put the ball into a 24x19 cm baking dish lined with baking paper and press mixture down to cover the bottom of the dish to form a good solid base.
7. Put in refrigerator, while you make the icing.

Icing Method

1. Put dates in bowl and just cover with hot water. Soak for 15 minutes.
2. Blitz cashew nuts in blender until very fine, remove from the blender.
3. Place dates and some date water in your blender and blitz to form a paste.

4. Add cashews, melted coconut oil, and melted cacao butter, to blender, and blend until smooth.
5. Add the rest of the ingredients and blend.
6. Pour icing onto base, and use a spatula to spread it out evenly.
7. Freeze for at least 10 minutes before cutting, then return to refrigerator to finish setting.

* Notes:

To melt cacao butter: place it in a small bowl and then sit the bowl in a larger container filled with boiling water, while you make the base. It should be melted in about 10 minutes.

If you prefer, you can substitute acai berry powder, or any other berry powder you like, for the maqui berry powder I used in this recipe. The choc fudge protein bar will keep in the refrigerator for up to 2 weeks, or it can be frozen to keep for longer periods.

NEXT Cacao Butter recipe:
| A7 | Cacao and Maca Latte | Pg.22

"Cacao is a well-known food source of magnesium, which is essential for healthy muscle and nerve function."

-Donna.

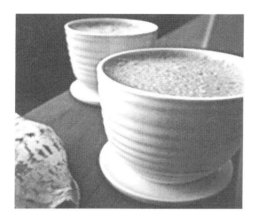

A7. Cacao and Maca Latte

Serving size: makes 1 cup
Time to make: 2 minutes

This cacao and maca latte will help you turn your back on coffee!

Ingredients

2 teaspoons cacao powder
1 teaspoon cacao butter
1 cup almond milk / or milk of your choice
1 teaspoon maca powder
¼ teaspoon vanilla paste / or dash of vanilla essence
1¼ teaspoons honey

Method

1. Place milk into pot on stove. When it's warm, add honey and vanilla paste. Whisk to mix.
2. Add cacao and maca powders and whisk again while it heats.
3. Be careful to remove from heat just before it boils.
4. Add cacao butter and whisk again while butter melts.
5. Then pour into a cup and enjoy.

* Notes:

TIP: Cacao butter holds heat - so be careful not to drink this latte too quickly.

If you have a milk 'frother' then you can use it to make your latte fluffy. Or aerate with a hand held stick blender or whisk to make your latte frothy to finish.

NEXT: Section B | Cacao Powder recipes | Pg.25

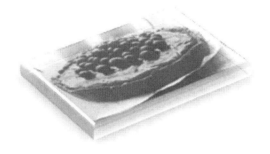

SECTION B

CACAO

POWDER

recipes

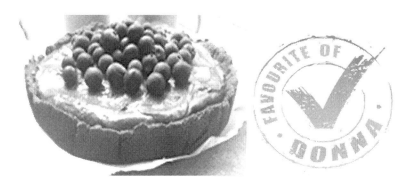

B1. Blueberry Chocolate Mousse Torte

Serving size: serves 8 -10 people
Time to make: 25 minutes

Base Ingredients

½ cup cacao powder
2 cups almond meal
⅓ cup lucuma powder
1 tablespoon maqui berry powder
½ cup melted coconut oil

Mousse Topping Ingredients

⅓ cup cacao powder
⅓ cup maple syrup
1 tablespoon maqui berry powder
½ teaspoon vanilla paste / or vanilla extract
¾ cup coconut cream
2 ripe avocados,
1 handful blueberries to garnish

Base Method

1. Combine the almond meal, cacao, lucuma and maqui berry

powders, with the melted coconut oil in a bowl. Mix with hands until it forms a large ball.

2. Press mixture firmly into the base of a 20cm flan tin. If the tin does not have a removable base, then line the tin with baking paper.

3. Chill base until set firm, in the refrigerator or freezer. This usually takes about 15 to 30 minutes.

Topping Method

1. Place the avocado, maple syrup, vanilla, cacao and maqui berry powders in a blender with the coconut cream and blitz until the consistency is smooth and well blended.

2. Spoon the mousse onto the chilled base, and place in refrigerator for 30 minutes, until the mousse sets.

3. When ready to serve, remove from tin and sprinkle a generous amount of blueberries on top.

* Notes:

This chocolate mousse torte is very quick to make and it really hits the spot! However, it is truly at its most delicious when eaten within 24 hrs of making, so don't hold back, enjoy it at its best.

NEXT Cacao Powder recipe:
| B2 | Cashew Nut Chocolate Ice-cream | Pg.28

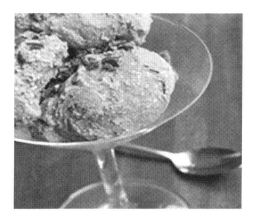

B2. Cashew Nut Chocolate Ice-cream

Serving size: 2 servings
Time to make: 10 minutes - excluding 2 hours soaking the cashews, and 1 hour in the freezer.

Ingredients

2 tablespoons cacao powder
1 cup cashew nuts - soaked for 2 hours, then drained
1 tablespoon vanilla extract
¼ cup coconut nectar / or yacon syrup / or maple syrup
1 pinch Himalayan salt
2 tablespoons lucuma powder
1 cup water / or milk, if you prefer
1 small sprinkle of cacao nibs

Method

1. Rinse soaked nuts and place in blender. Blitz nuts until well chopped, then add remaining ingredients and blitz all together.
2. When the mixture is well processed, pour into a shallow dish and place in the freezer.

3. Ready to eat after 1 hour in the freezer.
4. Garnish with a small sprinkle of cacao nibs and serve.
5. Enter ice-cream heaven.

* Notes:

TIP: The water content in this ice-cream makes it set very hard when frozen. The longer it is in the freezer the harder it will get, so you will need to allow your ice-cream to thaw a little bit before eating, or serve before it sets too hard.

NEXT Cacao Powder recipe:
| B3 | Chocolate Chia Pudding | Pg.30

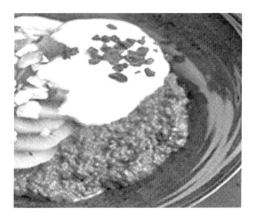

B3. Chocolate Chia Pudding

Serving size: Serves 1- 2
Time to make: 10 minutes (excluding 40 mins -1 hr standing time)

Ingredients

¼ cup chia seeds
1 cup almond milk
1 tablespoon cacao powder
1 tablespoon sacha inchi protein powder
1 teaspoon maqui berry / or acai berry powder
½ teaspoon vanilla paste / or vanilla essence

Method

1. Place chia seeds in a breakfast bowl.
2. In a separate bowl, combine all other ingredients and whisk with a hand held stick blender, or shake in a jar until combined.
3. Pour wet ingredients over chia seeds and stir till chia seeds sink. Or, swirl the bowl to make the chia seeds sink. Let the bowl stand for 10 minutes, then stir again.

4. Place pudding in fridge overnight, or let it stand for no less than 30 minutes and up to 1 hour, when it should be set and ready to eat.
5. Serve for breakfast with fresh fruit and coconut yoghurt. Drizzle with maple syrup and top with sliced almonds.

* Notes:

TIP: This breakfast is plant-based and protein-charged, so it can be more filling than it looks! Just letting you know.

NEXT Cacao Powder recipe:
| B4 | Rich Chocolate Mousse | Pg.32

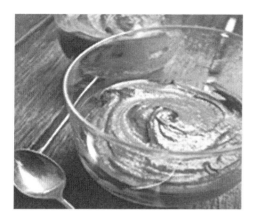

B4. Rich Chocolate Mousse

Serving size: serves 2
Time to make: 10 minutes

Ingredients

5 tablespoons cacao powder
3 tablespoons yacon powder / or lucuma powder
2 large avocados
¼ to ½ cup yacon syrup / or maple syrup / or honey
1 teaspoon vanilla extract
¼ cup water
1 pinch of salt

Method

1. Blend all ingredients together in the blender till well combined.
2. Spoon mixture into serving dishes.
3. Chill for a couple of hours and serve.

* Notes:

It is hard to believe this recipe is so quick and easy – but it is!

The chocolate mousse turns out really thick and creamy and you would never guess that it contains avocados - and *no dairy* at all.

I recommend using yacon powder and yacon syrup if you can, because I think that is the yummiest combination. But you should try the different combinations using lucuma powder, maple syrup, or honey, and see which you prefer.

NEXT Cacao Powder recipe:
| B5 | Gluten-free Chocolate Bliss Balls | Pg.34

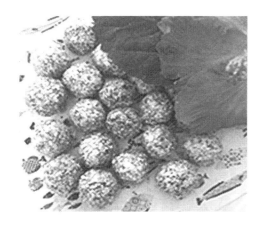

B5. Gluten-free Chocolate Bliss Balls

Serving size: makes about 18 small balls
Time to make: 30 minutes

Ingredients

2 tablespoons cacao powder
1 cup chopped dried apricots – try to find moist ones
¾ cup fresh medjool dates - chopped and with pips removed
1 cup chopped raw almonds - preferably activated
2 tablespoons coconut chips / or desiccated coconut
2 tablespoons chia seeds
2 tablespoons lucuma powder
1-2 tablespoons soft coconut oil
1 tablespoon liquid honey

Method

1. Place all ingredients in blender or food processor and blitz until well combined.
2. Adjust moisture, with honey and coconut oil.

3. Press into balls and roll in desiccated coconut / or cacao powder.
4. Refrigerate and grab when desired for a guilt-free treat.

* Notes:

My friend Suzie sent me this recipe; it is another of the delicious, gluten-free superfood treats that she seems to specialize in. I am fortunate to have such lovely and talented friends.

NEXT Cacao Powder recipe:
| B6 | Easy Chocolate Sauce | Pg.36

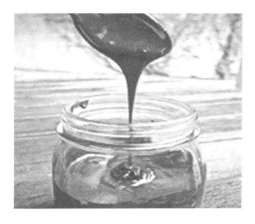

B6. Easy Chocolate Sauce

Serving size: makes 1½ cups
Time to make: 5 minutes

Ingredients

1 cup cacao powder
1 cup yacon syrup / or maple syrup
1½ tablespoons vanilla extract
3 tablespoons melted coconut oil
1 pinch of salt

Method

1. In a blender mix cacao powder, maple syrup, vanilla extract and salt until smooth. Slowly pour in the melted coconut oil while blender is still running.
2. When well blended pour chocolate sauce into a glass jar. Your chocolate sauce is now ready to eat, or store in the refrigerator.

* Notes:

Remember to remove your chocolate sauce from the refrigerator ahead of time, to allow sufficient time for the sauce to soften up *enough,* to allow it to pour easily.

I often sit the jar in some warm water for 5 minutes - which seems to soften the sauce perfectly. This easy chocolate sauce will store in the refrigerator for several weeks.

NEXT Cacao Powder recipe:
| B7 | Spicy Hot Chocolate Drink | Pg.38

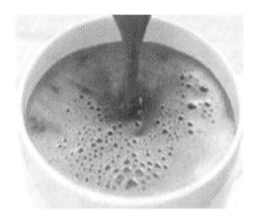

B7. Spicy Hot Chocolate Drink

Serving size: serves 2
Time to make: 5 minutes

This mood elevating spicy hot chocolate drink is just perfect for banishing the 'winter blues'. Just the mention of Hot Chocolate often sends calorie counters running for cover. However, this recipe is easy, and has loads of health benefits.

Ingredients

2 heaped teaspoons cacao powder
2 cups milk (milk of your choice, I prefer almond milk)
1 teaspoon lucuma powder
2 teaspoons coconut sugar / or honey (Note: coconut sugar has low G.I)
½ teaspoon cinnamon
1 pinch cayenne pepper (be careful – you only need a pinch)
1 teaspoon pure vanilla essence

Method

1. Heat milk in a saucepan, but don't let it actually boil. This is important, as it affects the *taste*.

2. Add all the other ingredients, cacao powder, lucuma, cinnamon, cayenne, coconut sugar, and vanilla. Whisk together until smooth.
3. Remove from heat. If you have a hand blender, you can aerate the hot chocolate to make it frothy before serving.
4. Pour into cups or bowls and indulge.

* Notes:

Cinnamon - is a warming stimulant, an astringent (contracts body tissues), is antiseptic and antiviral. It is traditionally used to aid digestive ailments such as flatulence, irritable bowel, nausea and diarrhoea.

Cayenne - is also a circulatory stimulant and cardiovascular tonic, apparently helping to reduce cholesterol and triglycerides. Historically it was used to increase blood-flow through the veins and arteries and increase a feeling of warmth.

NEXT: Section C | Cacao Nibs recipes | Pg.41

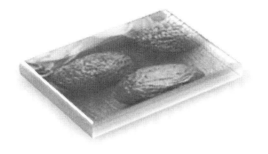

SECTION C

CACAO NIBS recipes

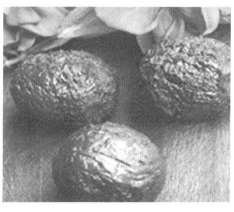
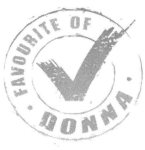

C1. Maqui Berry Cacao Truffles

Serving size: makes 16 Truffles
Time to make: 25 minutes

These maqui berry cacao truffles are packed with antioxidants and so easy to put together. They can also be served as a dessert.

Ingredients

2 tablespoons cacao nibs
2 tablespoons cacao powder
$\frac{1}{3}$ cup maqui berry powder
1½ tablespoons coconut oil
2 tablespoons lucuma powder / or yacon powder
1 tablespoon raw / or roasted smooth almond butter
1 cup packed soft medjool dates - pits removed / or dried dates soaked in warm water for 10 minutes.
1 dash sea salt

Method

1. Combine all ingredients except for the cacao nibs in a food processor, and process until a dense dough is formed.

2. Add the nibs and pulse a couple of times to combine, leaving in some textural crunch.

3. Roll one heaped teaspoon at a time into 1-inch balls.

4. Place on a plate and refrigerate for a minimum of 1 hour before serving. Always serve chilled or truffles will be too soft.

5. Optional: roll truffles in maqui berry powder on a plate, to dust exterior of the truffles before refrigerating.

* Notes:

This is a great recipe to have on-hand for an energising treat. The maqui berry flavour is delicious and it offers an extensive nutritional profile.

NEXT Cacao Nibs recipe:
C2 | 'Emergency' Ice-cream | Pg.44

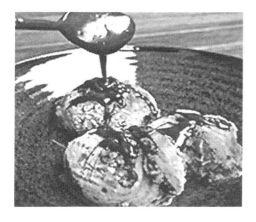

C2. 'Emergency' Ice-cream

Serving size: serves 2
Time to make: 5-10 minutes

This is 'the' ice-cream to reach for when you absolutely *must* have ice-cream! It is soooo good. Plus, it's quick, easy, and healthy too! That's crazy good news for you ice-cream fans out there.

Ingredients

½ cup cacao nibs
2 frozen bananas
1 cup frozen berries
2 tablespoons cacao powder
1 tablespoon blueberry powder / or you can use maqui berry powder / or acai berry powder
1 tablespoon maple syrup
1 teaspoon vanilla extract

Method

1. Place frozen bananas and berries into a sturdy blender and blitz until well chopped.
2. Add remaining ingredients to the blender and blitz again.

3. When suitably blended and the mixture is firm enough to be moulded, press into ice-cream balls and serve immediately, or store in freezer until required.

* Notes:

You can make this ice-cream even more delectable (if that's actually possible) by serving it with a drizzle of chocolate sauce (see 'Easy Chocolate Sauce' on pg.36 in Cacao Powder recipes, section B). However, it's still incredible eaten on its own.

TIP: Be sure to remove ice-cream from the freezer for a few minutes to soften before eating, as it freezes quite hard.

NEXT Cacao Nibs recipe:
| C3 | Delicious Chocolate Muffins | Pg.46

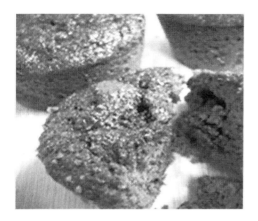

C3. Delicious Chocolate Muffins

Serving size: makes 12 muffins
Time to make: 30 minutes

Ingredients

4 tablespoons cacao nibs
1 cup almond flour
3 tablespoons coconut flour
1 teaspoon lecithin
1 tablespoon baking powder
3 tablespoons cacao powder
4 tablespoons honey
4 tablespoons melted butter
4 eggs
1 mashed banana
½ cup dried cranberries / or your choice of dried fruit

Method

1. In a bowl place all dry ingredients and mix together.
2. In another bowl beat 4 eggs, add melted butter and honey and add mashed banana.

3. Mix dry ingredients with wet ingredients.
4. Drop into paddy tins and bake at 160 degrees Celsius, for about 15 minutes.

* Notes:

My friend Debs, who often teams up with me as my partner at 'superfood demos', introduced me to this wonderful chocolate muffins recipe. She knows I'm not usually a muffin person, but she knew me well enough to know I'd like <u>these</u> ones.

I've 'played' with the original recipe a little, adding my own tweaks, so I must get Debs over soon for coffee and a batch of muffins and get her expert opinion on my version. We could even *pretend* we're working!

NEXT Cacao Nibs recipe:
| C4 | Anna's Chocolate Crunchies | Pg.48

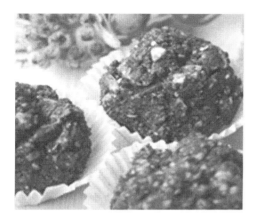

C4. Anna's Chocolate Crunchies

Serving size: makes 30 crunchies
Time to make: 30 minutes

Ingredients

¼ cup cacao nibs
2 cups coconut oil – somewhere between hard and runny
¾ cup cacao powder
¼ cup lucuma powder
1 tablespoon vanilla essence
½ cup maple syrup / or yacon syrup
1 cup chopped almonds
1 cup chopped walnuts
½ cup chopped pecans
½ cup sunflower seeds, toasted
¼ cup pumpkin seeds, toasted
1 cup shredded coconut

Method

1. Using a balloon whisk, beat coconut oil on medium speed
    until it becomes fluffy. Keep scraping sides as you go. Or you

can use a hand held beater. A food processor won't work because the mixture needs to be aerated. This only takes a minute or so.

2. Add cacao, lucuma, vanilla essence and maple syrup then blend until smooth.
3. Mix in other ingredients by hand.
4. Spoon into medium sized paper baking cases sitting in muffin tins.
5. Store in the refrigerator.

* Notes:

This chocolate 'crunchies' recipe was gifted to me by my friend, Anna. I have played with it a little bit, and you can too, according to your personal tastes and what you happen to have in your superfood pantry.

"They're delicious, and oh so healthy! I used the chocolate rice krispies (breakfast cereal) we had as kids as inspiration." - Anna Fairhall-Cate.

NEXT Cacao Nibs recipe:
C5 | Serious Protein Balls | Pg.50

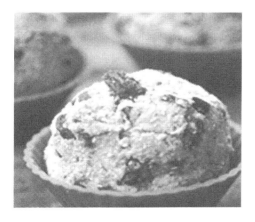

C5. Serious Protein Balls

Serving size: makes 10 balls
Time to make: 10 minutes

This recipe is quick and easy. It is for those wanting to increase their plant-based protein intake or have some on-hand for a post workout snack.

Ingredients

1 tablespoon cacao nibs
2 tablespoons coconut flour
3 teaspoons sacha inchi protein powder
1 tablespoon psyllium husks
½ cup coconut milk (may need a little more)
2 tablespoons maple syrup / or honey / or yacon syrup
1 tablespoon goji berries

Method

1. Place coconut flour, protein powder, psyllium husks in the blender with coconut milk and maple syrup.
2. Blitz until sticky (takes about a minute).

3. Add goji berries and cacao nibs by hand then squeeze into balls and place in refrigerator, or freezer, to set.

4. They are ready to eat after about 30 minutes.

* Notes:

At first, these ingredients don't look like they will 'bind' together, but the moisture *absorbing* quality of the coconut flour will allow this to happen after only a short time.

Serious Protein Balls will stay fresh for 3-4 days in the refrigerator.

NEXT Cacao Nibs recipe:
| C6 | Ancient Grains Fruit & Nut Bars | Pg.52

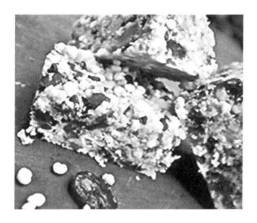

C6. Ancient Grains Fruit & Nut Bars

Serving size: makes 30 bars
Preparation time: 30 minutes

Ingredients

½ cup cacao nibs
1 cup puffed millet
1 cup flaked amaranth
½ cup chopped macadamia nuts
½ cup sultanas
¼ cup dried cranberries
¼ cup chopped dried apricots
¼ cup desiccated coconut
¼ cup sunflower seeds
1 teaspoon cinnamon
1 teaspoon ginger
6 tablespoons coconut oil
5 tablespoons peanut butter / or nut butter of your choice
3 tablespoons honey

Method

1.   Place all the dry ingredients and fruit in a bowl. Mix well.

2. Melt coconut oil, peanut butter and honey in a saucepan over very low heat. You only need to use heat until the coconut oil is melted.
3. Pour oil mixture over dry ingredients and mix well with a wooden spoon so that all ingredients are damp.
4. Press into dish lined with baking paper and place in your refrigerator to set.
5. Before it sets hard, cut into bar shapes and place back in refrigerator.

* Notes:

You can be creative with this recipe and substitute my dry ingredients for your favourites, or whatever you have available in your pantry. You can also add a heaped teaspoon of acai, blueberry, or maqui berry powder, if you have some.

NEXT Cacao Nibs recipe:
| C7 | Chocolate Smoothie 'pick-me-up' | Pg.54

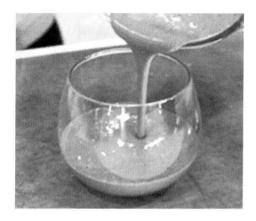

C7. Chocolate Smoothie 'pick-me-up'

Serving size: serves 1
Time to make: 5 minutes

This Chocolate Smoothie is my 'rescue remedy' for half-way through the afternoon - especially in summer-time when I often feel like I can't *last* until dinner time.

A delicious chocolate smoothie takes the emptiness away, as well as satisfying naughty taste-buds that are craving something totally *decadent*!

Ingredients

1 tablespoon cacao nibs
1 tablespoon cacao powder
1 tablespoon lucuma powder
1 frozen banana (skin off)
1 glass of almond milk / or milk/liquid of your choice
2 fresh medjool dates / or 2-3 dried dates soaked for
about 15 minutes in warm water
1 'small handful' of raw, pre-soaked almonds
1 tablespoon yacon syrup / or maple syrup

Method

1. Chop dates and add to blender with nuts, almond milk, chopped frozen banana, cacao powder, cacao nibs, lucuma powder and maple syrup.
2. Blend till smooth and creamy.
3. Serve in a tall glass and enjoy.

* Notes:

You can create your own variations on this basic chocolate smoothie by adding 1 or 2 of your favourite superfood ingredients each time you make it. Try adding maca powder or acai berry powder. If you don't have any raw almonds, try adding some sacha inchi protein powder instead.

The possibilities are endless, so enjoy creating your very own delicious chocolate smoothie to boost your energy and also be your own mood elevating 'rescue remedy.'

NEXT: Health Benefits of Cacao | Pg.56

Health Benefits of Cacao

Nature's raw, organic superfood chocolate ...

Cacao contains high levels of the antioxidants that are vital for protecting our cells and tissues from disease, and that may actually help to slow cell degeneration. Cacao is also rich in magnesium, iron, calcium and potassium.

The flavonoids in cacao powder have been the subject of many studies and it is currently believed they may contribute to the lowering of blood pressure and cholesterol, as well as assisting in cardiovascular health and the anti-aging process.

Phytochemicals such as epicatechins and procyanidins, as well as the alkaloid theobromine, all contribute to the nutritional prowess of the cacao bean and its derivative products such as cacao powder, cacao nibs and cacao butter.

Epicatechins, apart from being a powerful antioxidant, are being researched for their beneficial effect on vascular function and blood pressure levels. Procyanidins, also found in red wine, are noted for their contribution to reducing coronary heart disease.

Furthermore, theobromine has been used to treat high blood pressure and, like caffeine, is a heart stimulant but is easier on the central nervous system than caffeine.

Plus, give your mood a lift...

I saved the best news until last; raw, organic cacao is a great *mood elevator*. [Cue, Sade.] It can give you a much needed mood lift on a bleak winter's day, or when life seems to be handing you lemon after lemon.

Sitting down with a lovely cacao-based hot chocolate drink (like my Spicy Hot Chocolate recipe, on pg.38 in section B) can be just the boost you need to get you over the temporary 'blues' and back on-track for the day. The fact that I've jazzed it up with some other beneficial superfood ingredients will also add to the overall package of positivity that you're putting into your body.

Superfoods sceptics will say that there is no 'absolute proof' (yet) that putting all these good things into your body leads to better health in the long-run. My answer is, try it and see for yourself. Superfoods obtained from a reputable source are natural, nutrient-rich, and uncontaminated by chemicals and preservatives; unlike most of the stuff you consume every day from your local supermarket.

Mainstream medical professionals (apart from surgeons) mainly provide drug-based solutions to health problems, which come with long lists of potential side-effects and disclaimers. The bottom-line of the small print is usually that 'you are choosing to take this drug at your own risk' and, having been warned, don't think you can sue the drug company if it all goes horribly wrong.

My experience (supported by a wealth of anecdotal evidence) with superfoods is that I feel better, my brain seems to work better, and 2 serious medical conditions, that I couldn't find an answer for using traditional medicine, went away.

Of course, you need to approach superfoods (like anything else) in a balanced and sensible way. So, if one cacao hot chocolate drink makes you feel better, don't drink ten of them! It won't be 10 times better for you. In fact, it would be bad for you. Like abusing caffeine or alcohol. Common sense.

Having experienced both sides of the equation in trying to keep my brain and body healthy, I know which one I prefer. The natural approach works better for me.

Donna Davidson

- August, 2016.

* * *

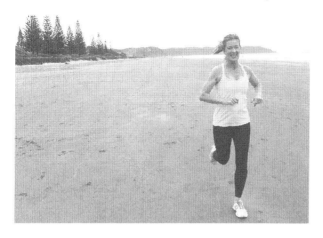

Donna Davidson Biography

- Author, business woman, recipe creator, 'superfoodie'.

Living happily by the Pacific Ocean, in New Zealand's beautiful North Island, Donna's primary passion has always been health, fitness and well-being.

Donna began her fitness career as an aerobics instructor; after receiving her diploma from Lords Gym in Perth, Australia, she trained at Jane Fonda's Workout Studio in Beverly Hills, California.

After establishing her own fitness studio back in Auckland, New Zealand, Donna was chosen to teach aerobics to New Zealand's Americas Cup yacht squad, as part of a new fitness and motivational program preparing them for their first Americas Cup challenge.

Later, while working in the superfoods industry, Donna experienced the profound benefits of adding superfoods to her regular diet. She now credits superfoods with helping her conquer 2 major health challenges in her life. Donna also realized that she had much more energy and increased mental acuity.

Wanting to share her discoveries with like-minded people, she decided to found her own superfoods company and online store; with the 'modest' aim of teaching as many people as possible about the benefits of superfoods, and making it easy for them to obtain them online.

The result was superfoodies.co.nz, which she created with the help of her friend, Kay Wood. Her goal was simple: to source the highest-quality superfood products and teach simple, sensible, delicious ways for ordinary folks to enjoy their health benefits. Without any hype or exaggeration.

Donna's first superfoods Kindle eBook, '21 Best Cacao (natural chocolate) Recipes' was launched in November, 2015 and quickly became an Amazon best seller - reaching the #1 spot several times!

The second book, '21 Best Superfood Smoothies', (in Donna's 'health through nutrition' themed 'Discover Superfoods' series) gives its reader 21 delicious ways to *drink* themselves to better health. It is also available to order online at Amazon.com as both Print book and Kindle eBook. (You don't need a Kindle device to download the eBook as they have free software viewers you can use on your computer or other device.)

Donna's third book, on 'Berry brain-foods' contains 21 of the best superfood berry recipes that can help us slow the ageing process and retain mental sharpness, as we get older. If you enjoyed this book, you'll definitely want to grab that one too. It is also available on Amazon. Hint, hint.

* * *

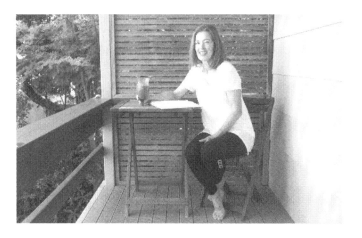

Donna's High Cholesterol story, in her own words ...

"Despite a strong sporting background and regular fitness regime, I still battled debilitating health issues earlier in my life, for which I couldn't seem to find an answer.

Quite by accident, the answer came when I landed a job in the superfoods industry; I experienced increasingly positive changes by adding specific superfoods to my daily diet.

I had been diagnosed with 'cyclic vomiting' syndrome. On average, once a month I would throw up for 24 hours, which just wiped me out physically. When I started having a green smoothie every morning this cycle soon completely disappeared.

I realized that my daily green smoothie was alkalising my digestive system and setting me up for the day. A second (unexpected) consequence was the rapid reduction of my bad cholesterol.

I have always been very fit and slim, so I had been totally shocked to find my cholesterol was at a dangerous level.

Although my mother had suffered from angina, and died with dangerously high cholesterol, aged 64, I had always considered myself 'fit and healthy' (despite my vomiting problem) and it had never occurred to me that I could be susceptible too.

After 3 months of drinking my green smoothie, my cholesterol went from 7.3 to 4.8. The result not only wowed *me*... but they *stunned* the nurse reading them out to me over the phone! I kept my printed test result sheets to prove to myself that I hadn't dreamt it, because even *I* couldn't believe it for ages. It took time to really sink in. I think, because it was literally life-changing for me.

To write the books in my 'Discover Superfoods' series meant I've had to draw deeply from all the knowledge I gained over 6 years of working in the superfoods industry, to create the best, easy-to-make, health-giving superfood recipes possible. These recipes will help you add loads of wonderful superfoods to your normal diet, in ways that are not just super nutritious and delicious, but often down-right decadent.

Please share your experiences with me, or ask me any question you may have. I'd love to hear from you."

Donna Davidson

- August, 2016.

* * *

FOLLOW - Donna on Facebook :: Facebook.com/SuperFoodies
EMAIL - Donna :: info@superfoodies.co.nz

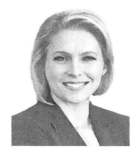
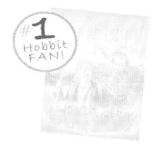

Kay Wood Biography

- Author, blogger, copywriter, web marketer, 'superfoodie'.

Originally from the world of advertising and marketing, Kay has more recently specialised in copywriting and content creation for the Internet. She also adores anything Tolkien, especially Hobbits.

For nearly 10 years Kay has been 'ghost-writing' info blogs for online businesses and offering her help to clients struggling to turn their awkward prose and bad spelling into simple and easily understood information about their products and services.

Kay and Donna became friends while working together to create Donna's superfoodies.co.nz website, in late 2013. Kay also worked closely with Donna to help her realise her ideas for the 'look and feel' of her superfood product packaging and the 'Superfoodies' logo design.

Kay and Donna found themselves 'clicking' as a team during that creative process. They both shared a common desire to present in an honest and balanced way the genuine health benefits to be gained by incorporating superfoods into one's diet - while at the same time dialling back some of the hype surrounding superfoods.

Kay's story, in her own words ...

"When I suggested to Donna that putting together some of her favourite and most delicious superfood recipes into a cookbook 'might be a good idea', to help show people how many ways superfoods can be incorporated into their diet, she initially hesitated because it sounded like such a daunting prospect to cover all, or even most, of the major superfoods in one book.

I later modified the original idea, suggesting to Donna that she should create a series of short, practical recipe books sharply focused on only one superfood in each book, pared down to the 21 absolute best recipes that Donna could come up with.

We both agreed that cacao would be the perfect superfood for book #1 - because everyone loves chocolate right? And healthy, or certainly healthier, ways to enjoy chocolate have got to be a great addition to any chocolate lover's recipe book collection.

So, with me cracking the whip and Donna creating, making, baking, eating and perfecting the recipes, this modest little book, 'Discover Superfoods #1: 21 Best Cacao Recipes' was born.

Try some of these wonderful cacao (natural organic chocolate) recipes for yourself, and I think you'll love them as much as we do!

Enjoyed in moderation, (for sadly, you can even eat too much organic chocolate) these 21 best cacao recipes will be a *lot* healthier, and better for you than the sugar and chemical-filled, commercial chocolate products at your local supermarket. But they still allow you to fully indulge your deepest chocolate desires; they are totally yummy.

Thanks, for buying our book! If you enjoy these recipes, please don't forget to give us a nice review on Amazon. That will really help us spread the good word to all those who still haven't heard that there are natural alternatives to junk food."

Kay Wood
- August, 2016.

Living in Aotearoa / New Zealand / Middle Earth - with the Hobbits.

What are Superfoods?

Superfoods are a special category of foods found in nature: these foods are superior sources of the essential nutrients and antioxidants that our bodies need, but cannot make themselves.

Superfoods are calorie-sparse and nutrient-dense, so they pack a lot of punch for their weight and deliver more of what our bodies need in one go. Foods that have been elevated to superfood status in recent years include those rich in antioxidants, vitamins, minerals, essential fatty acids, including omega-3 fatty acids.

Contrary to what some people wrongly believe, Superfoods are NOT nutrition created through advancements in food sciences. They are actually looking back to nature for what it does best: providing us with amazing and complex combinations of nutrients, beautifully balanced to supply us with what our bodies require to flourish.

This is simply going back to the wild and harnessing foods in their natural forms, with all their benefits intact. It is celebrating nature's wealth of nutrients in all its varieties. We have within our reach a true powerhouse of natural ingredients to provide us with the nutrition we need for healthy living.

Many superfoods are unique to their own geographical position in the world and this is usually because their local environment was perfect for producing them. Fortunately, in our modern world of advanced communication, travel and cultural appreciation, we are currently discovering an abundance of nutrient-rich superfoods we have previously never heard of. e.g. superfoods from South America, like the sacha inchi seeds, maqui berries, maca root, lucuma, and camu camu.

See Superfood Descriptions on pg.66 of this book, for more info.

There is no official definition of a superfood, and the EU has banned the use of the word on packaging, but that hasn't stopped many food brands from funding academics to research the health benefits of their products. Nor does it deter the health conscious from seeking and following eating regimes abundant with good nutrient-dense foods that they enjoy and feel the benefits of.

Superfoods can be processed under 40 degrees Celsius without damaging their nutritional profile and being classed as 'raw foods'. This makes storage and availability more convenient and versatile. e.g. superfood powders for smoothies and snacks are generally dried below 40 degrees Celsius.

An awareness of the kinds of foods that we're now calling 'superfoods', has been increasing rapidly over the last few years. Along with a better appreciation for how the foods we consume affect our bodies, as well as our long-term health.

We're also finding ourselves being 're-introduced' to many of the foods that were well-known to past generations, yet have been neglected for decades. We have lost touch with the knowledge of plants and natural compounds that our supposedly more primitive ancestors used to survive and heal themselves, before drugs were invented.

This is a knowledge that we all need to re-discover – if only to balance out the modern reliance on artificial drug based treatments. We're not saying that all drugs are bad, but returning to a lot of the effective yet natural ways of maintaining and restoring our health can't be a bad thing, either.

That way we can save drugs for serious health problems that require sudden, dramatic intervention. Thus, we may actually increase their efficacy and, by reducing their usage, also reduce the risk of creating drug resistant bacteria and the instances of harmful side-effects. Our immune systems will also thank us. Drugs often weaken our immune systems by killing the pro-biotic bacteria in our gut, interfering with the body's ability to digest food properly.

* * *

Superfoods Descriptions + Info

These are the dried superfoods Donna uses in her recipes:

Sacha Inchi protein powder: Vegetable protein powder from the South American Sacha Inchi seed. Contains 60% complete protein, all essential amino acids, as well as the omega essential fatty acids. Easily digestible and light nutty flavour. Perfect for pre/post workout smoothies, to maintain and build muscle.

More about Sacha Inchi powder + where to buy it :
Type into your web browser: www.superfoodies.co.nz/des-a

Maqui Berry powder: Reported to have the highest antioxidant/anthocyanin content than any other fruit or berry. Grows wild in the patagonian rain forests of Chile and Argentina. Contributes to cardiovascular health, cellular protection against oxidative stress, immune support and detoxification. Maqui berry powder is deep purple in colour and has a delicious rich berry flavour.

More about Maqui Berry powder + where to buy it :
Type into your web browser: www.superfoodies.co.nz/des-b

Acai Berry powder: Like maqui berry powder, acai has a very high antioxidant content with unique structures of anthocyanins for cellular protection and phytochemicals believed to lower cholesterol levels. Contains high levels of vitamin E and essential fatty acids to support clear smooth skin. Acai is low in sugar, deep purple in colour and perfect for smoothies and breakfast recipes.

More about Acai Berry powder + where to buy it :
Type into your web browser: www.superfoodies.co.nz/des-c

Lucuma powder: Comes from a fruit native to the Peruvian Andean region. It provides beta-carotene known for immune support as well as calcium phosphorous and iron for energy. It has a low glycaemic score of around 25 while it imparts a natural sweet, creamy, citrusy, maple flavour.

More about Lucuma powder + where to buy it :
Type into your web browser: www.superfoodies.co.nz/des-d

Maca powder: Contains unique alkaloids known to stimulate the hypothalamus and pituitary glands which in turn improve the overall functioning of the endocrine system responsible for balancing hormones. Grown in Bolivia and Peru it has a vanilla/nutty taste which is very appealing in smoothies. Although one of the most popular and consumed superfoods it is a food that can make some people feel queasy or have stomach cramps, but this is not common. I recommend small doses to start with e.g. 1 teaspoon in a smoothie, working up to 1 tablespoon per day.

More about Maca powder + where to buy it :
Type into your web browser: www.superfoodies.co.nz/des-e

Yacon powder: A natural sweetener containing high levels of inulin a fructooligosaccharide that provides sweetness in a form that is indigestible by humans so they do not affect blood sugar levels and simply pass through the digestive tract to be eliminated. Since these sugars are not digested and also low in calories they are suitable for use in diet and low calorie foods.

More about Yacon powder + where to buy it :
Type into your web browser: www.superfoodies.co.nz/des-f

Yacon syrup: The same as yacon powder, it's GI is only ONE. I find this syrup delicious in recipes, cacao drinks and smoothies. It is the perfect substitute for maple syrup if you are watching your sugar intake, often not easy to find and unfortunately a little more expensive.

More about Yacon syrup + where to buy it :
Type into your web browser: www.superfoodies.co.nz/des-g

Camu Camu berry powder: The camu camu berry from the Amazon region is presenting higher levels of vitamin C than any other fruit tested to date. Latest results are showing 56 times more vitamin C than Lemons. It is a potent addition for any smoothie.

More about Camu Camu berry powder + where to buy it :
Type into your web browser: www.superfoodies.co.nz/des-h

Blueberry powder: Well known for its antioxidants and anthocyanins. It also contains resveratrol also found in grapes which has been linked to heart health. A convenient powder to add flavour to smoothies.

More about Blueberry powder + where to buy it :
Type into your web browser: www.superfoodies.co.nz/des-i

Chia seeds: A must have ingredient for a superfood pantry. When added to smoothies they make you feel full and satisfied for longer periods.Chia seeds contain more omega 3 fatty acids than salmon. They are low glycaemic and are another source of protein.

More about Chia seeds + where to buy it :
Type into your web browser: www.superfoodies.co.nz/des-j

Fermented greens powder: A powerful formula which acts as a natural probiotic because of the good bacteria produced from the fermentation process. This natural probiotic aids digestion, assists absorption and has many healing functions. It is my personal MUST HAVE in a morning smoothie to set me up for the day.

More about Fermented greens powder + where to buy it :
Type into your web browser: www.superfoodies.co.nz/des-k

Cacao powder: Cacao powder has an extremely high antioxidant score on the ORAC scale. By eating high antioxidant foods in our diet it is believed we are helping to guard against cellular and tissue damage which often lead to serious illness.

Magnesium is abundant in Cacao Powder and it is magnesium that is known to be the most important mineral for a healthy heart. Cacao is a mood elevator due to the presence of serotonin.

More about Cacao powder + where to buy it :
Type into your web browser: www.superfoodies.co.nz/des-l

Cacao butter: Is the ingredient that sets chocolate and other chocolate treats. It contains oleic acid which is the same healthy fat found in olive oil. It also is a good source of vitamin E. It does not need to be stored in the refrigerator. It melts to liquid at 35 degrees Celsius.

More about Cacao butter + where to buy it :
Type into your web browser: www.superfoodies.co.nz/des-m

Cacao nibs: Has a similar nutritional profile to cacao powder. Nibs are the shavings and fragments from the cacao bean. They add crunch and texture to chocolate treats and smoothies.

More about Cacao nibs + where to buy it :
Type into your web browser: www.superfoodies.co.nz/des-n

* * *

Superfoods Testimonials

These are a few typical examples of unsolicited testimonials and comments about superfood products from happy customers who purchased from Donna's own website: superfoodies.co.nz

Lost over 7kg and feeling so much better …

"Thank you so much for the healthy delicious treats for Christmas. I am still enjoying my new eating regime with super foods. I have lost over 7kg and feeling so much better in myself. Everyone comments on how well I look and that my skin is glowing. Coming along to your sugar free cooking class was the best thing I have done in a long time." - **Kate.**

* * *

My husband is really noticing the benefits …

"Nick my husband has been using the green smoothie powder and really noticing the benefits – he is a landscaper so needs the energy - plus he has sinus problems and this has really helped with that as well. Brilliant." - **Annemarie.**

* * *

Helping me cope with the stresses of my current life …

"Still going strong with the smoothies and have one most days. Really like them and I think they are helping me cope with the stresses of my current life – very sick husband, work, coping with ten staff, visitors and the rest of the daily grind. They fill me up now that I add soy or almond milk until the next meal and I have found that my sweet tooth has dissipated to a large degree – not wanting something sweet every day, which is a real bonus. So all good, and all thanks to you!" - **Sigrid.**

* * *

I'm 'regular as clock-work' – without medication … wahoo!

"I'm pleased to tell you that I am having a smoothie every morning and my Green Smoothie Shot and the great thing is, I have been able to stop taking the Laxsol tablets that I have had to take for years. I decided to stop taking them straight away because they aren't life threatening (just uncomfortable if it didn't work) to see if the Chia seeds and Green Smoothie Shot made any difference immediately and I'm pleased to say it has, and I've never been able to go off these tablets before, so now I'm 'regular as clock-work' and without medication … wahoo!

Now for the extra good news, **I have lost 2kgs in just under 2 weeks** of using the Chia Seeds, Cacao Powder and Green Smoothie Shot - so the products are obviously cleansing my body well. I'm using all natural 100% pure coconut water in my smoothies and a frozen banana which is awesome." – **Michele.**

* * *

Immediately noticed an increase in my energy and general wellbeing …

"At last I can get a fermented probiotic greens powder (Donna's Green Smoothie Shot) in New Zealand! I have been searching high and low for a fermented greens powder in New Zealand since I moved here some years ago. When living in Sydney I was introduced to this product and I immediately noticed an increase in energy and general wellbeing – I was overworked and I truly think that this is what helped keep me going. When I left Australia I took as much with me as I could carry in my case, but that is long gone and I have been missing it ever since.

So thank you 'SuperFoodies.co.nz' for bringing this wonderful product to New Zealanders – it is every bit as good as I remember!" – **Xenia.**

* * *

I have already made <u>double-lot</u> of Choc Fudge protein bars …

"Thank you very much for yesterday, I so enjoyed it. Have already made 'double-lot' of Choc Fudge protein bars and my children like them!" – **Hiria Wallace.**

* * *

Enhanced our well-being and energy (and didn't get sick) …

"My husband and I have just returned from a month's trip around Morocco and every morning we took "Green Smoothie Shot" without fail. We were pleasantly surprised we did not experience any sickness and felt this product enhanced our well-being and energy to make the most of our holiday." – **Yvonne Porter.**

* * *

I learnt so much and changed my eating already …

"I learnt so much and have changed a few things with my eating already. Would love to carry on learning more." – **Jodeen Mitchell.**

* * *

You are so passionate about healthy food …

"Thanks ladies! You're both awesome. Very inspiring, as you are both so passionate about healthy food. Will try recipes out on my family – **Jeanette Pleijte.**

* * *

Read more Testimonials
superfoodies.co.nz/category/testimonials/

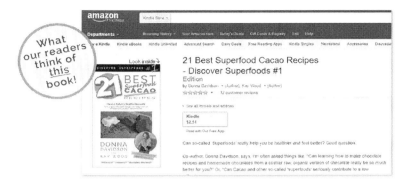

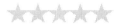

★★★★★ 5 Star Amazon Book Reviews:

- "Love Chocolate AND fitting into your Jeans? This book is for you."

- "I had a very different idea of what super foods were. Thank you."

- "Imagine the healthiest form of dessert you could possibly come by."

- "I have to confess... I didn't even make it through the whole book before I stopped to make one of the recipes!"

- "A Chocolate fanatic's must have!"

- "Quick, easy and delicious - an inspiring collection of superfood treats."

- "I think a craving for sweets is probably my biggest vice. The recipes in this book sound too good to be true, but having read the ingredient explanations, I really want to give them a try!"

- "I was impressed with the authors' explanation of how adding superfoods to our diet can help improve our overall health and provide much needed energy."

See more reviews here > www.amazon.com/dp/B0178USZ88

WHERE TO START?

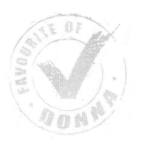

TRY ME!

Isn't 'fresh' always best?

And other Frequently Asked Questions, like:

1. What are all these superfood powders and dried processed products?
2. Isn't fresh always best?
3. What makes them 'super' foods - as opposed to ordinary foods?
4. How do these dried processed superfoods compare with fresh foods that are also called superfoods?
5. Are all these powders and dried stuff really superfoods?
6. Where can I get all these fancy dried superfood products?
7. Do they sell them in my local supermarket or do I have to go to a Health Food Shop?

* * *

If *you've* asked any of these questions, here are the answers, according to Donna and Kay:

QUESTION: "So, why are you using 'dried' superfood powders and products in these recipes?"

KAY'S ANSWER: This is something that often seems weird to people unfamiliar with using the dried forms of superfood products that are now available on the market.

In an ideal world, we would all have acai berries, maqui berries, blueberries, bananas, and cacao growing fresh in our backyards and we would pick them at the height of their potency and use them fresh every day.

Sadly, no matter where you live, this would be practically impossible. Either for climatic reasons, soil suitability, time poverty, lack of backyard garden space, lack of knowledge about how to actually grow and maintain these kinds of plants, and a zillion more reasons.

Even the supposedly 'fresh' fruits and vegetables we have available locally vary in nutritional value and taste, because of rising population numbers, they have to be grown quickly, picked, preserved, transported, displayed, and sometimes artificially enhanced to look appealing to consumers. The average 'fresh' tomato that most modern city dwellers eat is vastly different to the 'fresh' tomato that our grandparents or great-grandparents would have eaten. I remember my father growing tomatoes and strawberries in our small town New Zealand backyard and how 'gobsmack-ingly' delicious they were compared with the bland equivalents I purchase from the supermarkets these days.

When the population of the planet was relatively small, a mere 200 years ago, it was possible (at least theoretically) to grow enough food for the whole population of the world on the fertile farmland available, while also allowing enough time for excess land to lay 'fallow' for several years in order for the soil to recover the nutrients sucked out of it by the plants as they grew. That goodness, of course, was transferred to us when we ate those plants. Now, however, with farmland diminishing worldwide and poor farm and land management practices being common in many parts of the world, we already have less farmland available than is required to feed us all. This means that the land is being over utilised, the nutrients being stripped and never replaced, leading to less and less nutrients in the actual fruit and vegetables being grown on that land.

And then there's contamination from chemicals, such as fertilisers and pesticides, pollution, climate change, contamination from poor storage, unhealthy additives, and bad practices engaged in by unethical companies quite happy to put profit before their customers' health.

In an ideal world, 'fresh' would reign supreme. But in the real world, often the best we can do is combine 'fresh' (hopefully from the least contaminated sources) with high-quality dried nutrient sources - like the superfoods we recommend - in order to give our bodies and immune systems access to nutrients that aren't guaranteed to be in our food anymore.

If you live in a city, and especially if you have a busy, pressurised lifestyle, you probably don't have a garden, or the time to maintain one. My dad knew what nutrients his tomatoes needed and what kind of things were bad for them. Even though I ate his produce with glee, I never acquired his knowledge or skills and have never had much of a garden, sadly. Now, I wish I'd taken more notice and been more willing to learn from him.

I'm sure the same is true for many people, especially those younger than me; the whole idea of growing things yourself is a foreign concept. For some people even the idea of eating green things is foreign, and they think all food comes in packages that you heat up in a microwave. For those people, on a practical level, it would be much easier to throw some dried superfood ingredients into a blender, chop up a few available fruits or vegetables from the supermarket, and blend them all into a delicious smoothie in a couple of minutes, than to contemplate actually growing anything – never-mind having the land, plants or seeds, tools, fertilisers, knowledge and time to actually do it. Not to mention controlling pests, without risk to you, or the soil. Whoops, I mentioned it!

Is a tropical rainforest growing outside your window?

Many of the wonderful dried superfoods we use are only found in South America - probably because of the peculiarities of that climate and the evolution that occurred there in the isolation of the fertile tropical jungles. We think that buying superfoods from ethically responsible companies - who pick them 'fresh' at exactly the right moment, dry process them within an hour or two of being picked to lock in their nutrient content at its most potent - is a great way to access the tremendous nutrient value they contain.

Some still say, "You can get *everything* you need by eating fresh fruit and vegetables from the supermarket". If you read everything I wrote prior to this, and still believe that's a true statement, then you are entitled to your opinion. Donna and I would respectfully disagree with you. We have seen many people restore their health and well-being, as well as supporting their immune systems to fight and often eliminate stubborn health conditions. This is anecdotal evidence for sure, but, often, anecdotal evidence is only evidence waiting for science to catch up.

We can't guarantee that everybody who tries superfoods will experience the same results, but the same would be true if you visited the doctor and he recommended a course of treatment or certain medications. A doctor will never guarantee you anything. Also, try contacting the drug companies and see if they'll guarantee you that their products will work. Even the ones that have been supposedly approved and double-blind tested.

At the end of the day, as Donna and I often say, the 'proof is in the pudding' and you need to try something for a reasonable period of time and see if it works for you. Of course, you should do your 'due diligence'. Do as much research as you can, reference as much expert opinion as you can, try and find as much testimonial from those who have similar conditions to yourself and see what results they obtained, and then … you still end up with having to decide whether you will try them to see if they'll work for you.

This would be true of *anything*.

When Donna first tried green smoothies to see if they would help lower her high-cholesterol levels, a few years ago, she never expected them to eliminate her chronic 'cyclic vomiting' problem as well. That was a total surprise. Her life changed completely just because she added a green superfood smoothie every morning! There was no medical solution available at the time. The best she could do was to 'manage' the problem with injections of drugs.

My own experience is less dramatic: I was experiencing stomach pains and just feeling generally fatigued and unwell. When Donna sent me some 'green smoothie shot powder' which I added to a morning smoothie I came right within a week and have felt more balanced and that my stomach and digestion was working as it should. I don't feel queasy and nervous about my gut the way I previously did when it felt unstable and uncomfortable on a regular basis, despite the fact that my diet was comparatively healthy.

I hope my thoughts on the 'why' part of the "*why* do you use these kind of dried products?' question, has helped.

I'll let Donna explain her ideas of the pros and cons between 'fresh versus dried' superfoods, since she has much more expertise, not to mention experience, than me.

Kay Wood - August, 2016.

* * *

'Fresh' vs. 'Dried' Superfoods ...

QUESTION: "How do these dried, processed superfoods compare with fresh foods that are also called 'superfoods'?"

DONNA'S ANSWER: I personally believe in and work with both.

When I am time poor, I'm grateful to have my stash of dried superfoods in my pantry, so that I can whisk up a delicious and satisfying smoothie and be on my way to take on the day. When I have time to spare and have been fresh produce shopping I enjoy experimenting with produce in season mixed with my superfoods.

I know I can 'bank' on the variety of tastes and nutrition in dried superfoods, and they are as easy as having the stock in my pantry.

Fresh produce is not always at your fingertips, unless you have a prolific garden ... lucky you. So I say, you can 'have it all' by combining the use of dried and fresh (whatever's seasonally available).

Here are some 'Pros and Cons' for fresh versus dried superfoods.

Fresh is Best - when:

1. You know you are buying or gardening organically.

2. Your produce is harvested at its peak nutritional stage.
3. Your produce is stored in a cool place or refrigerator.

Downside of 'Fresh':

1. Using fresh produce requires lots of your 'TIME' for organisation, storage, planning, and preparation.
2. Seasonal unavailability of your favourites.

Dried is Best - when:

1. They are harvested at their nutritional peak and immediately processed to lock in their nutritional profile.
2. You can safely buy organic and see where the product is from on the label.
3. Storage is more convenient and takes up less space.
4. No produce preparation in the form of cutting, washing etc.
5. Less shopping.
6. Less planning ahead.
7. If you buy from a reputable company, quality and purity is more certain.

Downside of 'Dried':

1. Taste is the only real downside to dried superfoods.

The huge advantage of dried superfoods is that they're preserved at the highest level of nutrient potency and degrade very slowly when well stored... but they beat the taste of fresh seasonal produce.

'Fresh' is delicious and nutritious; offering a wide variety of taste and flavour combinations, depending on the season. Whenever I make a smoothie or design a recipe I never rely solely on the dried superfood products because, although they may be delivering the desired nutritional punch that our bodies and immune systems need so desperately, our taste buds also need to enjoy themselves!

That's why my recipes are full of 'real foods' and 'superfoods', in the forms of fresh fruits, nuts, seeds, and vegetables, as well as dried superfoods. I want the recipes to be a balance between taste and health, so they deliver on both fronts. In previous generations we often believed that if it was good for you it had to 'taste bad' - but these days we expect healthy food to be delicious and delightful to our taste buds, as well.

That's my goal when I sit down to design any new recipe. If I'm modifying an existing recipe, it will be because I can improve either the nutritional content, or the taste factor, or both. That was pretty easy for this book because it's all about chocolate recipes so they weren't too hard to make delicious, or healthy either - as long as you use good quality cacao (powder, nibs or butter). Make sure you stick closely to my recipes, though - don't be tempted to add any 'nasties' - like extra sugar - or you will undermine all my good work!

Sometimes, when you're beginning to add superfoods to your diet, your taste buds will need a little time to adjust to the lack of excess sugar and salt and other nasties that your system has been used to. Don't worry, after a very short time you will begin to enjoy the wonderful variety of natural flavours that were masked by these unhealthy additives in the past. *Then* your taste buds will begin to take you on a voyage of (re)discovery of flavours and taste sensations that you've been missing out on, or not enjoying to their fullest intensity.

Donna

- August, 2016.

* * *

Where can I get these 'dried' superfoods?

If you haven't heard of some of the superfoods (fresh or dried) – like lucuma powder or acai berries, for example - that Donna uses in her recipes, you may be wondering, "Where may I obtain these weird and wonderful new superfood ingredients?"

1. Health Food and Organic Stores
2. Pharmacies / Drug Stores
3. Specialty Food Shops
4. Some Supermarkets – ask at your local supermarket
5. Websites – order from local businesses online
6. Amazon.com – or your country's Amazon website
7. Google – search for stores and products nearest to you

Until relatively recently, superfoods - in any form - have been enjoyed mainly by a small niche market of fans who stumbled across them, or had them recommended by a friend or family member. In the last few years, more supermarkets have begun putting their toe in the water by offering a small line of dried superfood products, which often seem to be located in an obscure corner of the supermarket.

Slowly but surely, superfoods are entering the mainstream consciousness; most people have heard the word 'superfoods' on television, or mentioned somewhere, but they haven't tried them and are probably still sceptical. Even if they *are* contemplating trying superfoods, they may not know where to start.

Supermarkets that *do* carry a selection of dried superfoods, may not carry every single one of the ones that we use in our recipes, and you'll probably need to ask an assistant where they are.

Most of the products we use should be available in your local Health Food or Organic Store. Stocking of certain ones may differ according to local regional differences and tastes. We recommend, using your phonebook to ring around and check first, before you trudge around town. Most health food businesses have a website, and checking this out first will save you time and shoe leather.

Donna sells her own personally blended superfood products 'exclusively online' to New Zealand and Australian customers, and there are probably similar online superfood stores in your country or region. Google is your friend; just try typing in the name of the product you're looking for and your location and hopefully you'll find what you're looking for nearby.

Since Donna's business is solely based down-under, the high cost of shipping generally makes it impractical and prohibitive to offer her products further afield than New Zealand and Australia.

If you live in the US, we recommend ordering via Amazon.com, if you don't have a preferred local supplier. Amazon makes it very easy. If you are based in the USA, it makes sense because ALL of the products we use are available on Amazon. You can order from the comfort of your own home, and their shipping costs are very reasonable within the US.

To help you choose from Amazon's huge range, Donna has selected a comparable matching superfood product on Amazon that she believes to be highest quality equivalent to her own range*. (See pg. 66 – 'Superfoods Descriptions + Info')

* NOTE: Because we don't *control* these products, we can't guarantee the Amazon links will always remain valid in the future.

If you don't want to shop online and you don't find a good local supplier on your first try, it may be a matter of persevering until you come across one you like.

We hope this advice helps you find a reliable source of superfoods locally. If not, reach out to us on Facebook and we'll try to help.

* * *

Conclusion

Try our 'Chocolate Pudding Challenge'...

Let's re-visit the question we posed at the start of this book, "Will 'superfoods' really help me be healthier and feel better?"

It is a good question. So, what's our answer?

It's tempting just to say, YES, they worked for me! But, for a more 'nutrient-dense' answer, let's look a little deeper at the quality of the food produced by our 'modern' food production methods.

Let's consider the vital relationship between our modern diet and our health. The steady and observable decline in health and rise of chronic conditions such as allergies, asthma, and skin conditions in western countries over the last 60-100 years is generally agreed by scientists and medical experts to be in large part attributable to changes in our diet.

What about other factors, like exercise?

The other biggest factor in this decline is undoubtedly the increasing trend of employment moving from outdoor, physical work to more sedentary occupations.

This takes us away from the natural source of vitamin D (the sun) and exposure to rare but necessary elements such as selenium (from soil); this trend not only weakens our muscles (including the heart) it also weakens our immune system (from lack of exposure to bacterial challenges) and slows our metabolism, decreasing its efficiency in burning up fats and other elements in our food that would, under our previous more vigorous outdoor lifestyle, have been burned up, utilised or expelled more quickly by our bodies.

Can it all be attributed to our modern lifestyle?

Combine the factors we touched on in the previous paragraph with the fact that our lungs (with subsequent flow-on to our blood streams) are now more likely to be sucking stale, unhealthy air (often) full of mould spores and germs into our bodies - rather than fresh air - on a regular basis, and you can see that our modern lifestyle is far less healthy than that of our grandparents or great-grandparents.

They probably worked outside and ate a lot of fresh, uncontaminated produce that they grew themselves, or at least had easy access to, in a way that most modern city-dwellers do not. What most modern city-dwellers *do* have easy access to, are lots of highly processed, packaged, nutrient-poor foods; full of added sugars, salts and fats; coloured and chemically enhanced to 'look' fresh. Yum, yum.

Ironically, advancements in medicine are keeping increasingly unhealthy, chronically sick people alive longer, to enjoy a poorer quality of life. That's our very broad overview of the modern diet and lifestyle in most 'western' countries; it seems to us to be becoming the reality for more and more people every day.

Thanks to the Internet, a growing awareness of these issues is spreading around the world and is leading to the strong realisation that we need to change our unhealthy eating lifestyles. We believe the rapid growth of the superfood community worldwide is also evidence of that. Unfortunately, *cost* shuts many out from healthier food and nutrition alternatives, including superfoods.

We've noticed the use of 'hype' in the marketing of certain 'trendy' superfoods…

Sadly, there are always some greedy or unscrupulous (or maybe even a few genuine, but ignorant) marketers who are willing to make extravagant claims around a particular 'currently trendy' superfood, in order to exploit the gullible, the vulnerable, and sometimes desperate people hoping for some miraculous cure for a serious health condition.

While superfoods can be helpful to many health conditions and will support the body in its fight to repair and heal itself, they're best used long-term as part of a healthy lifestyle and balanced diet, for general health. They are unlikely to produce a miraculous effect on someone in the last stages of a major or life-threatening illness. Please consult your licensed medical practitioner for advice if you, or a loved one, are thinking of incorporating superfoods as part of a treatment program for any such condition.

However, for most people, there are many compelling reasons to consider adding superfoods to your diet. While sceptics remain, it is hard to deny the increasing wealth of anecdotal evidence for the benefits of incorporating superfoods into one's diet.

On the simple principle of 'rubbish in, rubbish out' it logically makes sense that putting natural, raw, organic foods into our bodies will generally lead to a better functioning bodily system than consuming nutrient-poor, non-natural foods full of chemicals and additives, as well as added sugars and fats.

The Superfood trend reveals…

There is an emerging awareness among like-minded people who are choosing to eat better, think better and feel better by eating healthy, nutrient-rich foods. These are the people Donna has dubbed 'superfoodies'; she coined this term to describe those who both love and are very knowledgeable about good food (foodies), but who also consider superfoods among the wisest and best ingredients to incorporate into the creation of good food.

* * *

Try our 'Chocolate Pudding' Challenge ...

Isn't the proof *always* in the pudding?

So, why not give superfoods a try?

In our experience, most people find, after adding superfoods to their regular diet (often by simply replacing breakfast with a superfood smoothie), that they feel more energetic; they start noticing improvements in, or even the total elimination of, minor health irritations; that they're losing weight, or maintaining a healthy weight; and generally feeling more sustained and balanced.

Elsewhere in this book we've included some of the testimonials and stories (See pg.70) that Donna gets regularly from people using her 'Superfoodies' products. You can find tons of completely independent testimonials if you Google, 'testimonials about superfoods' (for example), to find loads more people reporting similar superfoods experiences all around the world.

You'll find all 21 recipes in this book delicious and easy-to-make, as well as being good for you and your loved ones.

We hope you enjoy them *all* and find yourself reaping the healthy rewards of superfoods, very soon.

Donna & Kay

PS. Don't forget you're not alone; there's a whole community of 'super foodies' travelling with you.

Please reach out to us via Facebook or email, if you need help making the recipes, or any other superfoods advice. We look forward to hearing about your journey.

Follow Donna :: on Facebook.com/SuperFoodies

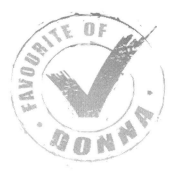

Still not sure which recipe to try first?

We recommend you start with one of Donna's
'Top 3 Tick Start' recipes. They're the
ones with this 'tick' icon.

They're on these pages:

Why not try one tonight?

Just *before* you rush off to the kitchen …

The End

Except

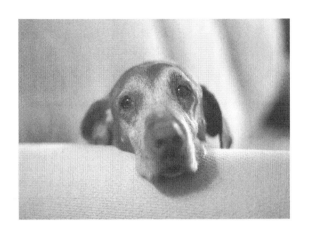

To thank *you* sincerely for buying our book!

We really appreciate it.

Would you be kind enough to help us make our next book *even* better ?

Please take 5 precious minutes to give us your honest REVIEW on Amazon.com

Thanks so much!

Donna & Kay

Recipe Diary

Have superfood fun being 'experimental'...

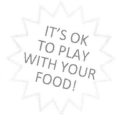

IT'S OK TO PLAY WITH YOUR FOOD!

Why this Recipe Diary?

Donna's recipes are designed around a base of 'core' ingredients that she has carefully balanced to deliver *nutritional punch* and flavour. They are intentionally built from a combination of 'dried superfoods' and healthy fresh ingredients that allow you to experiment around these core ingredients, to create your own variations, adapting each recipe to your own personal tastes.

* Note: Smoothie recipes are great to adapt because, ideally, you'll be using them a lot so it's good to have alternatives for variety and when there is seasonal un-availability of certain fresh ingredients.

One day, Donna intends to release a book which specifically isolates the (absolutely essential) *core* ingredients in her recipes and highlighting which *optional* ingredients may be exchanged with others; without losing any of the targeted benefits and nutritional value.

But until that book comes out, why not conduct your own experiments to see what variations on Donna's recipes will work for you? Obviously, not *every* ingredient change will work, so you may have a misfire or two, but that's all part of the fun!

Donna does a lot of *experimenting* herself, and brings a lot of existing knowledge and years of experience to guide her, but balancing nutritional content with appropriate flavour combinations can be tricky sometimes. That's why 'tried and true' combinations are great starting points. Sometimes you may have to compromise on one thing in order to retain another. Some great flavour combinations are not necessarily as healthy or beneficial as others that may be less agreeable to the taste buds. The ideal result, of course, is to achieve the perfect balance of both.

Since Donna has done most of the work with these recipes, she recommends that you try your own experiments to find out if your own personal favourite will work - once you've given the originals a fair go, of course!

The best way to do this would be to change out only *one* of the fresh ingredients each time you make the recipe, and see what you think. Is it good? Does it taste terrible? Does it work with the other ingredients? Once you think you're on the right track, you could try adding one or two more new flavours with additional fresh ingredients. Don't forget to try some nuts or seeds, too.

Donna recommends you don't go 'overboard' with adding 'too many' new ingredients, because your body can only absorb so many good things in one go. You may be just wasting your money, time - and ingredients. That's why it's best to start with one change, then proceed up to two or three in total. If your experiments work, that will give you sufficient new options, without going crazy!

There will also be plenty of times when adaption, or experimentation, is absolutely necessary!

Sometimes this will be forced upon you by seasonal un-availability of fresh fruit and vegetables, or by the fact you simply forgot to replenish your pantry! It happens to the best of us. You've been busy rushing around all week and finally that birthday party or gathering of family or friends is suddenly upon you. You planned to delight everybody with your amazingly healthy chocolate treats, but when you rush to the pantry... shock, horror!... some key ingredient of a recipe is missing! Maybe more than one. You've got literally, 'no time' to replenish them, so you're forced to adapt and try to find something new to replace what is missing.

That's a great reason, for trying a few 'experiments', with ingredient variations, long *before* you find yourself in that dire situation.

It's not such a daunting prospect if you already *know* that certain flavour combinations are successful, and you already understand how to 'balance' different flavour 'profiles' against each other. 'Tried and true' is only that way because, back down the track, someone tried experimenting until they got it right! You don't want find yourself experimenting on your guests, and hoping it's not a disaster!

So, after you've given the existing recipes a good and thorough try-out (which should keep you busy for a while), use these Diary pages to keep track of your 'experiments'. Record the details here.

Don't just rely on your memory, especially in a moment of panic. It's much better to come back to your notes, in your very own handwriting, in this section of the book, and confirm what your memory is telling you.

How to use this Recipe Diary:

1. Have Fun by Experimenting with Donna's Recipes.

2. Record the results in this Recipe Diary.

3. Change-out <u>one</u> of the recipe ingredients (fresh is easiest).

4. If you like the new change, either stop there or continue.

5. Add/change, up to 2 more additional ingredients.

6. Record your changes, and thoughts on the results in 'Notes'.

7. Rate your Experiment out of 7, and then circle either:
Yes – No – Maybe.

Go and have lots of fun. Happy experimenting!

Experiment #1

Recipe Notes:

Don't rely on your memory! Fill in *all* the details here and you'll always know exactly what you did - and if it worked or not.

Date: ....

Recipe Name: ....…........

Change #1: ....

Change #2: ....

Change #3: ....

*My Results: ....

....

....

....

Rate the Result: [Circle the number you believe to be the fairest.]

| 1 | 2 | 3 | 4 | 5 | 6 | 7 |

* <u>Don't</u> forget to record what you learn about different flavour combos. Could the new flavour work in a different recipe, or combination? Could it work with the addition of a balancing flavour/or flavours? If any other *inspired* ideas occur as you go, note them down for future experiments.

Circle one: YES!   NO!   MAYBE?

Experiment #2

Recipe Notes:

Don't rely on your memory! Fill in *all* the details here and you'll always know exactly what you did - and if it worked or not.

Date: ....

Recipe Name: ....…......

Change #1: ....

Change #2: ....

Change #3: ....

*My Results: ....

....

....

Rate the Result: [Circle the number you believe to be the fairest.]

| 1 | 2 | 3 | 4 | 5 | 6 | 7 |

* <u>Don't</u> forget to record what you learn about different flavour combos. Could the new flavour work in a different recipe, or combination? Could it work with the addition of a balancing flavour/or flavours? If any other *inspired* ideas occur as you go, note them down for future experiments.

Circle one: YES!   NO!   MAYBE?

Experiment #3

Recipe Notes:

Don't rely on your memory! Fill in *all* the details here and you'll always know exactly what you did - and if it worked or not.

Date: ....

Recipe Name: ....

Change #1: _____

Change #2: _____

Change #3: _____

*My Results: _____

_____

_____

_____

Rate the Result: [Circle the number you believe to be the fairest.]

| 1 | 2 | 3 | 4 | 5 | 6 | 7 |

* <u>Don't</u> forget to record what you learn about different flavour combos. Could the new flavour work in a different recipe, or combination? Could it work with the addition of a balancing flavour/or flavours? If any other *inspired* ideas occur as you go, note them down for future experiments.

Circle one: YES!   NO!   MAYBE?

Experiment #4

Recipe Notes:

Don't rely on your memory! Fill in *all* the details here and you'll always know exactly what you did - and if it worked or not.

Date: ....

Recipe Name: ....

Change #1:

Change #2:

Change #3:

*My Results:

Rate the Result: [Circle the number you believe to be the fairest.]

1   2   3   4   5   6   7

* Don't forget to record what you learn about different flavour combos. Could the new flavour work in a different recipe, or combination? Could it work with the addition of a balancing flavour/or flavours? If any other *inspired* ideas occur as you go, note them down for future experiments.

Circle one: YES!   NO!   MAYBE?

Experiment #5

Recipe Notes:

Don't rely on your memory! Fill in *all* the details here and you'll always know exactly what you did - and if it worked or not.

Date: ....

Recipe Name: ....

Change #1: ....

Change #2: ....

Change #3: ....

*My Results: ....

Rate the Result: [Circle the number you believe to be the fairest.]

| 1 | 2 | 3 | 4 | 5 | 6 | 7 |

* <u>Don't</u> forget to record what you learn about different flavour combos. Could the new flavour work in a different recipe, or combination? Could it work with the addition of a balancing flavour/or flavours? If any other *inspired* ideas occur as you go, note them down for future experiments.

Circle one: YES!   NO!   MAYBE?

Experiment #6

Recipe Notes:

Don't rely on your memory! Fill in *all* the details here and you'll always know exactly what you did - and if it worked or not.

Date: ....

Recipe Name: ....….......

Change #1:

Change #2:

Change #3:

*My Results:

Rate the Result: [Circle the number you believe to be the fairest.]

1   2   3   4   5   6   7

* <u>Don't</u> forget to record what you learn about different flavour combos. Could the new flavour work in a different recipe, or combination? Could it work with the addition of a balancing flavour/or flavours? If any other *inspired* ideas occur as you go, note them down for future experiments.

Circle one: YES!   NO!   MAYBE?

Experiment #7

Recipe Notes:

Don't rely on your memory! Fill in *all* the details here and you'll always know exactly what you did - and if it worked or not.

Date: ....

Recipe Name: ....…........

Change #1: _____

Change #2: _____

Change #3: _____

*My Results: _____

_____

_____

_____

Rate the Result: [Circle the number you believe to be the fairest.]

| 1 | 2 | 3 | 4 | 5 | 6 | 7 |

* <u>Don't</u> forget to record what you learn about different flavour combos. Could the new flavour work in a different recipe, or combination? Could it work with the addition of a balancing flavour/or flavours? If any other *inspired* ideas occur as you go, note them down for future experiments.

Circle one: YES!   NO!   MAYBE?

Experiment #8

Recipe Notes:

Don't rely on your memory! Fill in *all* the details here and you'll always know exactly what you did - and if it worked or not.

Date: ....

Recipe Name: ....……

Change #1:

Change #2:

Change #3:

*My Results:

Rate the Result: [Circle the number you believe to be the fairest.]

1   2   3   4   5   6   7

* <u>Don't</u> forget to record what you learn about different flavour combos. Could the new flavour work in a different recipe, or combination? Could it work with the addition of a balancing flavour/or flavours? If any other *inspired* ideas occur as you go, note them down for future experiments.

Circle one: YES!   NO!   MAYBE?

Experiment #9

Recipe Notes:

Don't rely on your memory! Fill in *all* the details here and you'll always know exactly what you did - and if it worked or not.

Date: ....

Recipe Name: ....…......

Change #1: _____

Change #2: _____

Change #3: _____

*My Results: _____

_____

_____

_____

Rate the Result: [Circle the number you believe to be the fairest.]

| 1 | 2 | 3 | 4 | 5 | 6 | 7 |

* <u>Don't</u> forget to record what you learn about different flavour combos. Could the new flavour work in a different recipe, or combination? Could it work with the addition of a balancing flavour/or flavours? If any other *inspired* ideas occur as you go, note them down for future experiments.

Circle one: YES!   NO!   MAYBE?

Experiment #10

Recipe Notes:

Don't rely on your memory! Fill in *all* the details here and you'll always know exactly what you did - and if it worked or not.

Date: ....

Recipe Name: ....

Change #1: _____

Change #2: _____

Change #3: _____

*My Results: _____

_____

_____

Rate the Result: [Circle the number you believe to be the fairest.]

| 1 | 2 | 3 | 4 | 5 | 6 | 7 |

* <u>Don't</u> forget to record what you learn about different flavour combos. Could the new flavour work in a different recipe, or combination? Could it work with the addition of a balancing flavour/or flavours? If any other *inspired* ideas occur as you go, note them down for future experiments.

Circle one: YES!   NO!   MAYBE?

Experiment #11

Recipe Notes:

Don't rely on your memory! Fill in *all* the details here and you'll always know exactly what you did - and if it worked or not.

Date: ....

Recipe Name: ....

Change #1:

Change #2:

Change #3:

*My Results:

Rate the Result: [Circle the number you believe to be the fairest.]

1   2   3   4   5   6   7

* <u>Don't</u> forget to record what you learn about different flavour combos. Could the new flavour work in a different recipe, or combination? Could it work with the addition of a balancing flavour/or flavours? If any other *inspired* ideas occur as you go, note them down for future experiments.

Circle one: YES!   NO!   MAYBE?

Experiment #12

Recipe Notes:

Don't rely on your memory! Fill in *all* the details here and you'll always know exactly what you did - and if it worked or not.

Date: ....

Recipe Name: ....…......

Change #1:

Change #2:

Change #3:

*My Results:

Rate the Result: [Circle the number you believe to be the fairest.]

1   2   3   4   5   6   7

* <u>Don't</u> forget to record what you learn about different flavour combos. Could the new flavour work in a different recipe, or combination? Could it work with the addition of a balancing flavour/or flavours? If any other *inspired* ideas occur as you go, note them down for future experiments.

Circle one: YES!   NO!   MAYBE?

Experiment #13

Recipe Notes:

Don't rely on your memory! Fill in *all* the details here and you'll always know exactly what you did - and if it worked or not.

Date: ....

Recipe Name: ....

Change #1: ....

Change #2: ....

Change #3: ....

*My Results: ....

Rate the Result: [Circle the number you believe to be the fairest.]

| 1 | 2 | 3 | 4 | 5 | 6 | 7 |

* <u>Don't</u> forget to record what you learn about different flavour combos. Could the new flavour work in a different recipe, or combination? Could it work with the addition of a balancing flavour/or flavours? If any other *inspired* ideas occur as you go, note them down for future experiments.

Circle one: YES!   NO!   MAYBE?

Experiment #14

Recipe Notes:

Don't rely on your memory! Fill in *all* the details here and you'll
always know exactly what you did - and if it worked or not.

Date: ....

Recipe Name: ....

Change #1:

Change #2:

Change #3:

*My Results:

Rate the Result: [Circle the number you believe to be the fairest.]

1 2 3 4 5 6 7

* Don't forget to record what you learn about different flavour combos.
Could the new flavour work in a different recipe, or combination? Could
it work with the addition of a balancing flavour/or flavours? If any other
inspired ideas occur as you go, note them down for future experiments.

Circle one: YES!   NO!   MAYBE?

Experiment #15

Recipe Notes:

Don't rely on your memory! Fill in *all* the details here and you'll always know exactly what you did - and if it worked or not.

Date: ....

Recipe Name: ....

Change #1: ....

Change #2: ....

Change #3: ....

*My Results: ....

....

....

....

Rate the Result: [Circle the number you believe to be the fairest.]

| 1 | 2 | 3 | 4 | 5 | 6 | 7 |

* <u>Don't</u> forget to record what you learn about different flavour combos. Could the new flavour work in a different recipe, or combination? Could it work with the addition of a balancing flavour/or flavours? If any other *inspired* ideas occur as you go, note them down for future experiments.

Circle one: YES!   NO!   MAYBE?

Experiment #16

Recipe Notes:

Don't rely on your memory! Fill in *all* the details here and you'll always know exactly what you did - and if it worked or not.

Date: ....

Recipe Name: ....

Change #1:

Change #2:

Change #3:

*My Results:

Rate the Result: [Circle the number you believe to be the fairest.]

1   2   3   4   5   6   7

* Don't forget to record what you learn about different flavour combos. Could the new flavour work in a different recipe, or combination? Could it work with the addition of a balancing flavour/or flavours? If any other *inspired* ideas occur as you go, note them down for future experiments.

Circle one: YES!   NO!   MAYBE?

Experiment #17

Recipe Notes:

Don't rely on your memory! Fill in *all* the details here and you'll always know exactly what you did - and if it worked or not.

Date: ....

Recipe Name: ....

Change #1: _____

Change #2: _____

Change #3: _____

*My Results: _____

_____

_____

_____

Rate the Result: [Circle the number you believe to be the fairest.]

| 1 | 2 | 3 | 4 | 5 | 6 | 7 |

* <u>Don't</u> forget to record what you learn about different flavour combos. Could the new flavour work in a different recipe, or combination? Could it work with the addition of a balancing flavour/or flavours? If any other *inspired* ideas occur as you go, note them down for future experiments.

Circle one: YES!   NO!   MAYBE?

Experiment #18

Recipe Notes:

Don't rely on your memory! Fill in *all* the details here and you'll always know exactly what you did - and if it worked or not.

Date: ....

Recipe Name: ....

Change #1:

Change #2:

Change #3:

*My Results:

Rate the Result: [Circle the number you believe to be the fairest.]

1   2   3   4   5   6   7

* <u>Don't</u> forget to record what you learn about different flavour combos. Could the new flavour work in a different recipe, or combination? Could it work with the addition of a balancing flavour/or flavours? If any other *inspired* ideas occur as you go, note them down for future experiments.

Circle one: YES!   NO!   MAYBE?

Experiment #19

Recipe Notes:

Don't rely on your memory! Fill in *all* the details here and you'll always know exactly what you did - and if it worked or not.

Date: ....

Recipe Name: ....…........

Change #1: ....

Change #2: ....

Change #3: ....

*My Results: ....

....

....

....

Rate the Result: [Circle the number you believe to be the fairest.]

| 1 | 2 | 3 | 4 | 5 | 6 | 7 |

* <u>Don't</u> forget to record what you learn about different flavour combos. Could the new flavour work in a different recipe, or combination? Could it work with the addition of a balancing flavour/or flavours? If any other *inspired* ideas occur as you go, note them down for future experiments.

Circle one: YES!   NO!   MAYBE?

Experiment #20

Recipe Notes:

Don't rely on your memory! Fill in *all* the details here and you'll always know exactly what you did - and if it worked or not.

Date: ....

Recipe Name: ....…........

Change #1: _____

Change #2: _____

Change #3: _____

*My Results: _____

_____

_____

_____

Rate the Result: [Circle the number you believe to be the fairest.]

| 1 | 2 | 3 | 4 | 5 | 6 | 7 |

* <u>Don't</u> forget to record what you learn about different flavour combos. Could the new flavour work in a different recipe, or combination? Could it work with the addition of a balancing flavour/or flavours? If any other *inspired* ideas occur as you go, note them down for future experiments.

Circle one: YES!   NO!   MAYBE?

Experiment #21

Recipe Notes:

Don't rely on your memory! Fill in *all* the details here and you'll always know exactly what you did - and if it worked or not.

Date: ....

Recipe Name: ....…..……

Change #1: ....

Change #2: ....

Change #3: ....

*My Results: ....

....

....

....

Rate the Result: [Circle the number you believe to be the fairest.]

| 1 | 2 | 3 | 4 | 5 | 6 | 7 |

* <u>Don't</u> forget to record what you learn about different flavour combos. Could the new flavour work in a different recipe, or combination? Could it work with the addition of a balancing flavour/or flavours? If any other *inspired* ideas occur as you go, note them down for future experiments.

Circle one: YES!   NO!   MAYBE?

Donna Davidson and Kay Wood

118

Don't forget...

1. Your <u>Free</u> Bonus: 3 Smoothie Recipes!

Type this into your Internet browser >
www.superfoodies.co.nz/ book1free

2. Our other Amazon books.

Book #2: '21 Best Superfood Smoothie Recipes'
Go here > www.amazon.com/dp/B01J73OAKG

Book #3: '21 Best Brain-food Berry Recipes'
Go here > www.amazon.com/dp/B01LWJLKOD

3. Please help us – with a totally honest <u>Review</u>.

We write our books with *you* in mind. Please take 5 minutes to give us your honest REVIEW on Amazon. Tell us what you <u>like</u> about our book(s) – and where we can <u>improve</u> for you, in future editions.

Review here > www.amazon.com/dp/B0178USZ88

Still turning pages?

Why?

Are you expecting a big …

Surprise!

AN EXTRA
BONUS RECIPE...

From Book #3 – '21 Best Berry Brain-food Recipes'
Out now on Amazon.com

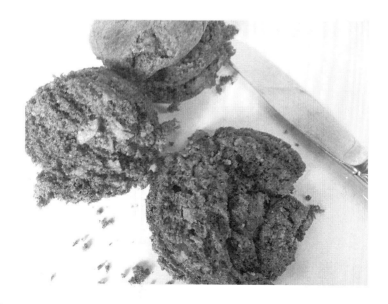

Boysenberry Muffins

Serving size: makes 6 large muffins
Time to make: 10 minutes prep + 35 minutes cook time

Ingredients

1 cup boysenberries

½ raw apple - finely chopped

1 tablespoon lucuma powder

2 teaspoons maqui berry powder / or acai berry powder

1 teaspoon cinnamon

1 teaspoon lecithin (optional)

1-2 teaspoons baking powder

1½ cups almond meal

1 pinch of salt

2 eggs

30 ml melted coconut oil

1 tablespoon honey / or maple syrup

Method .

1. Heat oven to 170C / 300F
2. Place all dry ingredients in a large mixing bowl.
3. Add coconut oil, honey and eggs.
4. Mix to a smooth batter.
5. Fold in berries and apple.
6. Spoon into 6 paper cups / or patty tins.
7. Bake in oven for 35 -40 minutes.

* Notes:

These boysenberry muffins are light and moist to eat, high in protein and are antioxidant rich. They may be the healthiest muffins you've ever eaten. They taste pretty good too!

* * *

[This recipe is from Book #3 – '21 Best Berry Brain-food Recipes'
- ORDERS: Kindle and Print versions now available on *Amazon.com*]

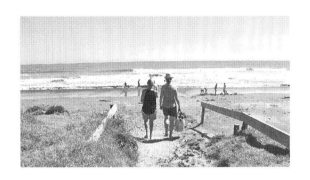

Bye, for now,

We're off to the beach.
See you in our next book.

-Donna & Kay.

:: End ::

Books by Donna & Kay

The Discover Superfoods Series – *by* Donna Davidson and Kay Wood.

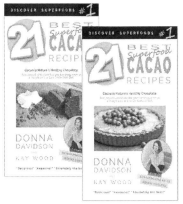

KINDLE / eBook
Discover Superfoods Book #1
21 Best Superfood Cacao Recipes
Available on Amazon.

PRINT BOOK
Discover Superfoods Book #1
21 Best Superfood Cacao Recipes
Available on Amazon.

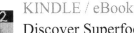

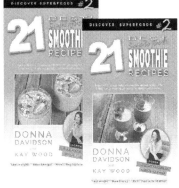

KINDLE / eBook
Discover Superfoods Book #2
21 Best Superfood Smoothie Recipes
Available on Amazon

PRINT BOOK
Discover Superfoods Book #2
21 Best Superfood Smoothie Recipes
Available on Amazon

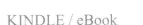

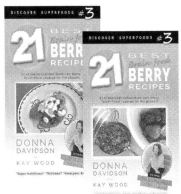

KINDLE / eBook
Discover Superfoods Book #3
21 Best Berry Brain-food Recipes
Available on Amazon

PRINT BOOK
Discover Superfoods Book #3
21 Best Berry Brain-food Recipes
Available on Amazon

The Secret
to better health?

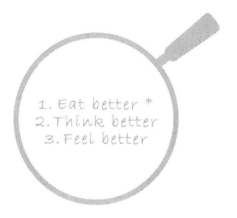

1. Eat better *
2. Think better
3. Feel better

* "Good food is better _medicine_ than medicine. If you enjoy the privilege of being able to choose
to eat better, you are among the lucky ones. Make that choice today and save
on your future medical bills, mental anguish, physical pain, and years
of living with a lower quality of life than you needed to."

– D&K.

Made in the USA
Lexington, KY
04 August 2019